A Los Angeles Bouncer's Guide to
Practical Fighting

A Los Angeles Bouncer's Guide to
Practical Fighting

by
Noah Knapp

Turtle Press   Santa Fe

A LOS ANGELES BOUNCER'S GUIDE TO PRACTICAL FIGHTING
Copyright © 2007 Noah Knapp. All rights reserved. Printed in the United States of America. No part of this book may be reproduced without written permission except in the case of brief quotations embodied in articles or reviews. For information, address Turtle Press, PO Box 34010, Santa Fe NM 87594-4010.

To contact the author or to order additional copies of this book call 1-800-778-8785 or visit www.TurtlePress.com

ISBN 978-1-880336-97-7
LCCN 2007036184
Printed in the United States of America

10 9 8 7 6 5 4 3 2 1 0

Warning-Disclaimer

This book is designed to provide information on martial arts and self-defense skills It is not the purpose of this book to reprint all the information that is otherwise available to the author, publisher, printer or distributors, but instead to compliment, amplify and supplement other texts. You are urged to read all available material, learn as much as you wish about the subjects covered in this book and tailor the information to your individual needs. Anyone practicing the skills presented in this book should be physically capable to do so and have the permission of a licensed physician before participating in this activity or any physical activity.

Every effort has been made to make this book as complete and accurate as possible. However, there may be mistakes, both typographical and in content. Therefore, this text should be used only as a general guide and not the ultimate source of information on the subjects presented here in this book on sambo or any skill or subject. The purpose of this book is to provide information and entertain. The author, publisher, printer and distributors shall neither have liability nor responsibility to any person or entity with respect to loss or damages caused, or alleged to have been caused, directly or indirectly, by the information contained in this book.

Library of Congress Cataloguing in Publication Data

Knapp, Noah.
 A Los Angeles bouncer's guide to practical fighting / by Noah Knapp.
   p. cm.
 ISBN 978-1-880336-97-7
 1. Self-defense. I. Title.
 GV1111.K58 2007
 613.6'6--dc22
                    2007036184

Special Thanks to:

Master Kishore Hiranand

Dan Biales

Dave Bradley

Carolina Hiranand

Wade Garrett

CONTENTS

INTRODUCTION 9

CHAPTER 1: STRIKE ZONES 11
    Proper Positioning 12
    Self Readying 13
    Diamond Point Fighting 15

CHAPTER 2: HAND AND ARM ATTACKS 21
    Proper Striking Area 23
    Hand Attacks 24
        Whole Fist 24
        Half Fist 26
        Backfist 28
        Knuckle Fist 30
        Star Fist/Eagle's Beak 32
        Finger Gouge 34
        Thumb Spike 36
        Palm Strike 38
        Claw 40
        Whip Hand Attack 42
        Knife Hand 44
        Chop 46
    Arm Attacks 48
        Wrist Attack 48
        Forearm Attack 50
    Elbow Strikes 52
        Obtuse Elbow Strike 52
        Acute Elbow Strike 54

CHAPTER 3: UPPER BODY MANIPULATIONS 57
    Mirror Hand 58
    Cross Hand 59
    3 Point Rolling Fists 61
        3 Point Outside Rolling Fists 61
        3 Point Inside Rolling Fists 63
        3 Point Upward Rolling Fists 65
        3 Point Downward Rolling Fists 67
        3 Point Destruction Rolling Fists 69
    4 Point Rolling Fists 70
        4 Point Outside Rolling Fists 70
        4 Point Inside Rolling Fists 72
        4 Point Bridge (Upward) Rolling Fists 74
        4 Point Downward Rolling Fists 76
        4 Point Destruction Rolling Fists 78
    Tunneling 80
        Double Hand Tunneling 81
        Single Hand Entry 84
        Forward Pullback 86

Spreading Waves		88
Kick separation	91	
Push Separation	92	
Bump Separation	93	

CHAPTER 4: FOOT AND LEG ATTACKS — 95
Proper Kicking Areas of the Foot		96
Kicks		99
Front Kick	99	
Check Kick	101	
Back Kick	102	
Side Kick	104	
Knee Attacks		106
High-Level Knee Attack	106	
Low-Level Knee Attack	108	

CHAPTER 5: LOWER BODY DEFENSE — 109
High-Level Leg Attacks	111
Mid-Level Leg Attacks	113
Low-Level Leg Attacks	121

CHAPTER 6: LOCKS, GRAPPLING AND FREEING — 123
Headlocks		124
Forward Facing Headlock	126	
Backward Facing Headlock	127	
Full Nelson	130	
Double Handed Choke	132	
Body Locks		134
Bear Hug	134	
Wrist & Arm Locks		136
Arm Bar (Defensive)	136	
Arm Bar (Offensive)	138	
Wrist Grabs		140
Cross-handed wrist grab	140	
Mirror Handed Wrist Grab	142	
Quick Change Wrist Grab (High)	144	
Quick Change Wrist Grab (Low)	145	

CHAPTER 7: STEPPING, TRAPPING AND SWEEPS — 147
Stepping & Trapping		148
Sweeps		149
Cross Leg Sweep	149	
Mirror Leg Sweep	152	

CHAPTER 8: READING YOUR OPPONENT — 155
Preemptive Movement	156
Stances	159
Guarding Postures	161

INTRODUCTION

First things first. This is an instructional guide on fighting, it will not show you how to do forms or one style perfectly; no martial art can or will be mastered from reading a book. However, the information within these pages will give you a clear understanding of and insight into realistic fighting tactics. For over 24 years I have trained and taught in many different styles of martial arts, including having ranked as a 3rd degree black sash in a survivalist style of Kung Fu, but it was truly my time as a bouncer in many of L.A.'s top night clubs that gave me the opportunity to see, first hand, which techniques work and which do not. This same knowledge, the knowledge that will make you a more complete and formidable adversary, is contained in the pages that follow.

Defending oneself at the onset of an altercation does not have to be an anxious or unsure time. With proper training and preparation, the possibility of bodily injury can be all but removed. Previous training in martial arts, boxing, etc. will definitely give one an advantage over their aggressor, however having an arsenal of seemingly limitless techniques usually does little more than leave one using up precious time guessing which will serve them best at the crucial moment. Most of the experienced martial artists that I have known readily admit to using only a small portion of the moves that were part of their training. Knowing this to be a common truth, I have compiled a list of techniques that have proven themselves extremely effective during my own personal combat. Every one of these moves is simple enough for beginners, but also sophisticated enough to compel even the most seasoned fighters.

This book contains only honest and realistic, although sometimes graphic self-defense techniques. Survivalist styles of kung fu teach swift, decisive movement that renders your opponent defeated in the fastest possible manner. Unlike the many "sport-style" martial arts, survivalist kung fu does not allow for the idea of "clean fighting." Rules have no place in real combat. Knowing kung fu's graphic applications, one of my students long ago asked me what to do if I didn't need to hurt my adversary to the fullest extent of my ability. My answer was only that if I didn't need to do my utmost, then I didn't need to fight at all. Get out quick and get out alive; those were my only goals. If I have learned anything during my time as a bouncer, it is only how true this lesson is.

INTRODUCTION

I have worked in some of the busiest and most popular spots in the Los Angeles nightclub scene and over many years I have been attacked with knives, lead pipes, guns and many other weapons, not to mention the countless occasions of hand-to-hand combat. I quickly learned to utilize my experience as a kung fu instructor to negate the advantage that any violent aggressor(s) could have over me. Having experienced far more than my fair share of conflict during this time, I had no choice but to refine my close-quarter techniques to the point where they were both extremely easy to perform and undeniably effective in their usage.

However confident in style or self, any experienced defense instructor will tell you that the most important thing to remember during any training is that your body comes first, not your ego. Taking upon yourself any risk in the mindset of just "striking your opponent harder than they can hit you" is never acceptable. What good is landing a devastating blow if your aggressor has just had the chance to do the same? Patience serves every fighter well and opportunities have more chance of occurring the longer you stay on your feet. Bodily safety comes first, no exceptions.

Having said this, try to consider that one of the most important skills a fighter can master is knowing what not to do. The purpose of this guide is not only to educate in a proactive manner, but also to inform the reader on the myriad of mistakes that fighters regularly fall victim to. In truth, most of the fights I have witnessed ended due to completely avoidable and headstrong mistakes on someone's part. But foolishness in defense is only one side of the story. Wasted strikes, unbalanced standing, ineffective blocking and risk of bodily injury have claimed more than one fighter over the years. All of these blunders can easily be eradicated by the simple lessons in each chapter. Important to consider is that the moves presented are not set in stone, but rather must be approached from the mindset that they can be changed on the fly so that they may still be used in realistic and unpredictable fights as well as just in training.

Every section analyzes both offensive and defensive possibilities. Used as a whole, this guide will prepare you to be at your best on either front. Remove your mistakes and you have removed your risk. Recognize your opponent's mistakes and you have removed their chance of any success. Either or both can easily eliminate the threat and win the fight.

CHAPTER 1
STRIKE ZONES

Any zone of the human body can be exploited in the pursuit of self-defense. However, just hitting someone where they are open has many times proven to be not enough. The mid-section of the body is filled with dozens of nerve points and sensitive areas, but these are worthless unless you know how to attack them. Landing a good open-hand attack on your assailant's stomach may not be the best of choices. Regardless of how hard you hit, the result will usually turn out to be no worse for your opponent than a good belly-flop in the local swimming pool.

The purpose of this chapter is to instruct on proper and effective offensive techniques and more importantly to aid in the removal of common mistakes. Far more times than I care to remember, I witnessed new bouncers on my security team throwing wild punches, hoping to win the lottery by landing a well placed shot; rarely if ever did this happen during such a situation. More often the result left them standing with no concept of protecting their own positioning and soon waiting to be rescued by their co-workers.

The first part of this chapter introduces the concept of readying and proper positioning. In this section, we cover the external zones of the body and which is the most effective manner to protect them. This will include both why, and how to maintain defense. The second part of this chapter hones in on the proper entries to striking zones of our opponent's body, not only concentrating on the "where" of but once again the "how to" aspect of obtaining and attacking them as well.

Proper Positioning

Observing proper posture is essential whenever any confrontation happens. Just as it will be possible to exploit your opponent's weaknesses, so it is also possible for another person to exploit your own. Proper posture removes not only your assailant's advantages, but also limits any offensive onslaught possibilities.

No matter the strength, size, or skill level of the person attacking, you must consider that your own upper hand is only one well-placed attack away. However, to allow for that opportunity to happen, you must first survive your opponent's attack. Listed below are the "do's" and "do not do's" of posturing and ready stances.

One of, if not the most foolish things I have ever seen in training is a ready stance that turns the shoulders sideways from your opponent in order to hide or conceal the centerline. It has been long understood that the centerline of the human body contains several kill zones that should be protected at all costs. However true this precaution is, in turning your shoulders to accomplish this task you have now rendered yourself completely exposed on another, just as important, zone of the body: the spine. You need only circle your hands in front of your eyes, throat, heart, stomach, and groin to see that your arms are well equipped to cover the area with ease. Try the same over the base of your skull, neck and spine and you will clearly understand why exposing even slight traces of your back is dangerous.

A safe and effective readying of your body is simply to place your hands forward in a "ward off position" and drop one foot slightly back while giving a small bend to your knees. Making sure to keep both shoulders forward and elbows bent, turn your toes inward to avoid a break from a quick kick and you find yourself in one of the most easily defensible positions ever conceived.

Proper Ward Off Positioning

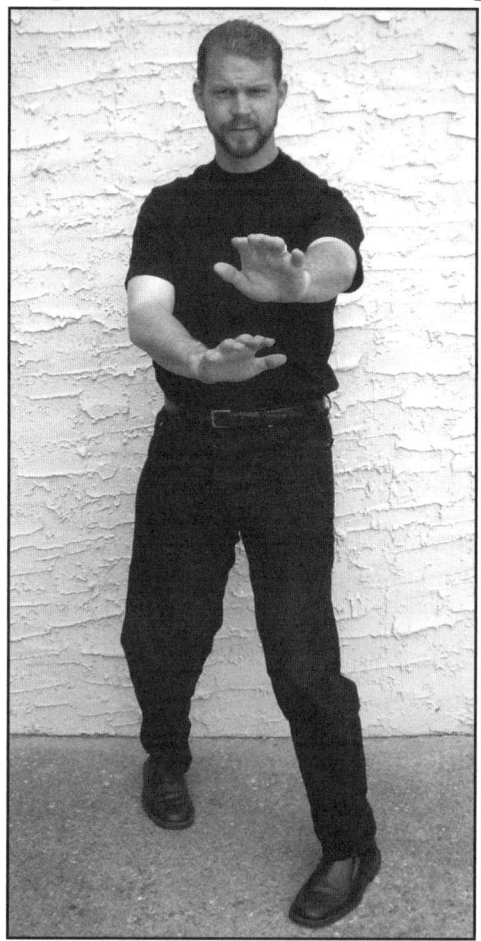

WARD OFF POSITION

Once in your ready stance, bear in mind one other factor. Whether defending or attacking, always keep your body as relaxed as possible with a slight bend in **all** joints. It is much more difficult to hyper-extend a bent joint than a joint that has already been prepared straight. Bent joints also offer quite a bit more in the realm of force absorption.

I have heard a thousand arguments about the added strength and effectiveness of a locked elbow and wrist during a punch. I have also exploited similarly locked joints too many times to recall. The fact of the matter is, one punch, no matter how effective it may be, is never worth the risk of personal injury. Better is the risk of less strength than that of a broken elbow or wrist.

Self Readying

Before physical contact is ever made, one must be aware of the area surrounding the body. An experienced fighter observes their surroundings the moment an altercation becomes a possibility. Some of the best fighters that I have ever seen have found themselves victims of their own ignorance, never considering that additional assailants may be only feet away. Bouncers regularly rely on this foolishness, distracting the rowdy patron's attention forward until addition members of the security team can take them by surprise from behind. It is unfortunate that all too often new bouncers try to brave it out and handle many altercations solo. However, the Queensbury rules don't apply when you are being attacked by a drunk whose best friend sees him losing harshly to your calm and sober mind.

Consider also simply walking down the street. Muggers regularly work in pairs. You may be surrounded and not even know it. Anyone who lives in a major city knows to keep their eyes open when they are out and about, but few realize how easy effective observation can be. Working in nightclubs forces one to learn these lessons quickly. Any bouncer hoping to make it past hour one of their first shift learns to instantly scan the area before engaging their opponent. A speedy and reliable way to assess your personal situation is to recognize "diamond points."

Diamond Point Fighting

Utilizing diamond fighting is possibly the easiest and most effective manner with which one can maintain their personal safely. The near perimeter around the body is best considered by recognizing the shape of a diamond with yourself standing in the center (below). The zone straight ahead of you is diamond point 1. At your right is diamond point 2. Diamond point 3 is directly behind. This leaves diamond point 4 at your left.

Diamond Point Positions

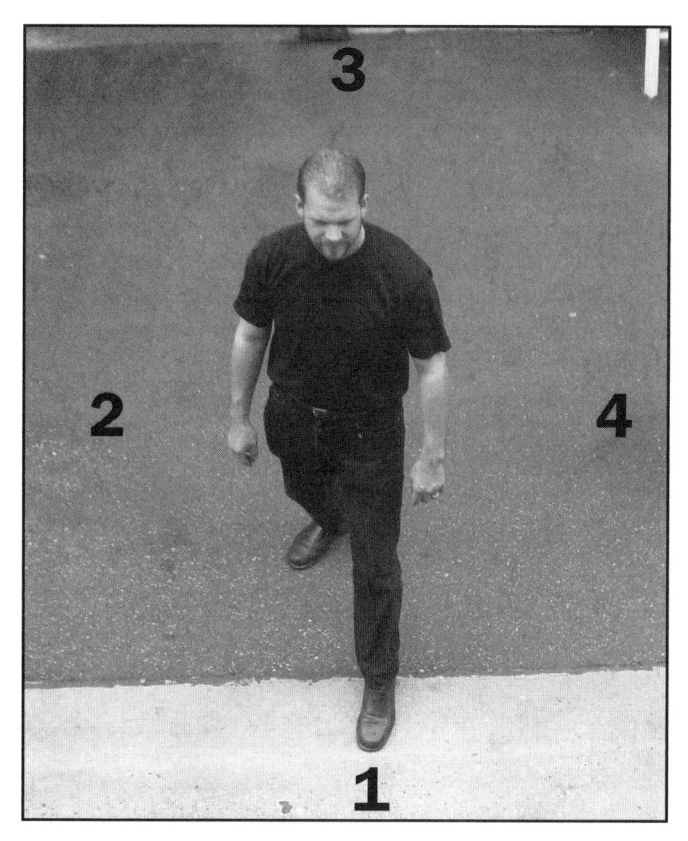

Scanning the area well for assailants will greatly increase your chances of success, but it is not only other attackers you should keep your eyes open for. Many other physical restrictions may exist, such as walls, tables, chairs, random wet spots on the floor, or even other non-aggressive persons. Any one of these can cause loss of control and should be considered before allowing an altercation to proceed. It takes only a split second to analyze the area around you.

Once your assets and limitations are determined, you will be left with a clear picture of the remaining safe avenues of escape surrounding you. Remember, you are only looking for best the possible path of free movement. Generalizing the four main areas surrounding you (diamond pts. 1-4) as viable or non-viable will give you a greater chance of success. Consider the following example:

Diamond Point Sequence

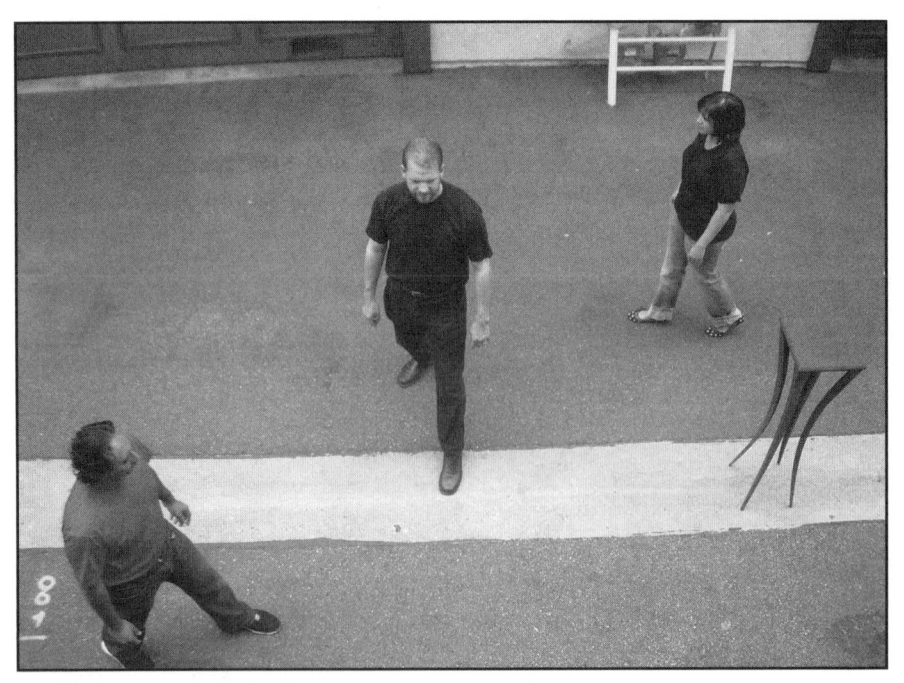

1. - YOU ENTER INTO A POSSIBLY HOSTILE SITUATION.

STRIKE ZONES

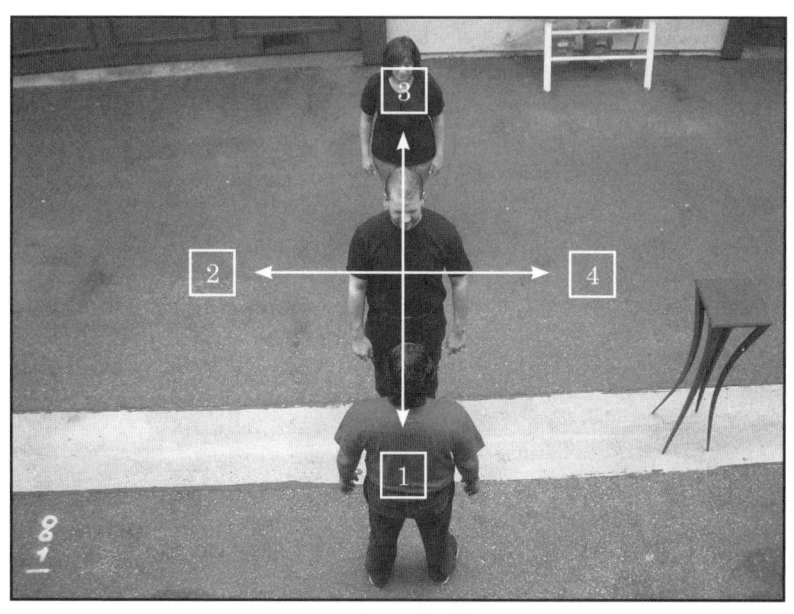

2. You confirm that your opponent has aggressive intentions.

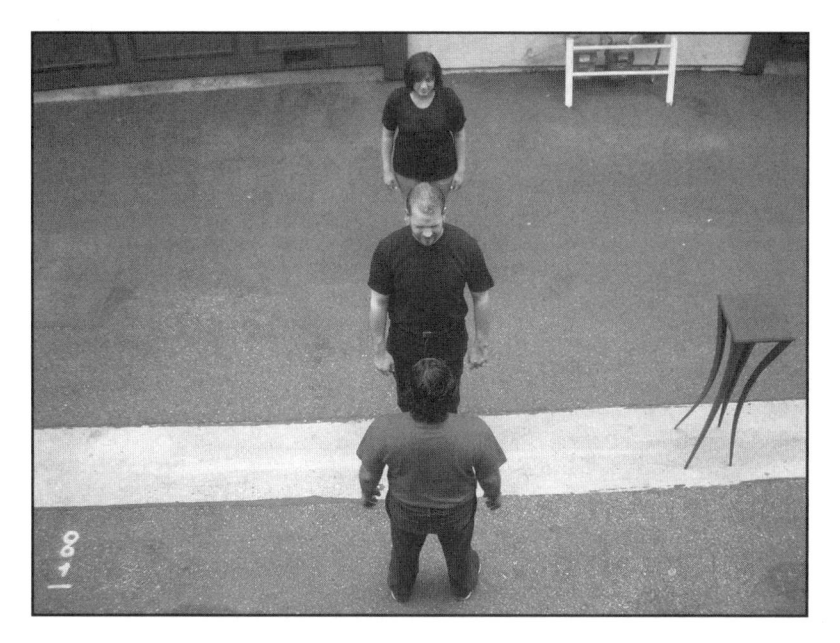

3. Quickly observe the four Diamond Points.

STRIKE ZONES

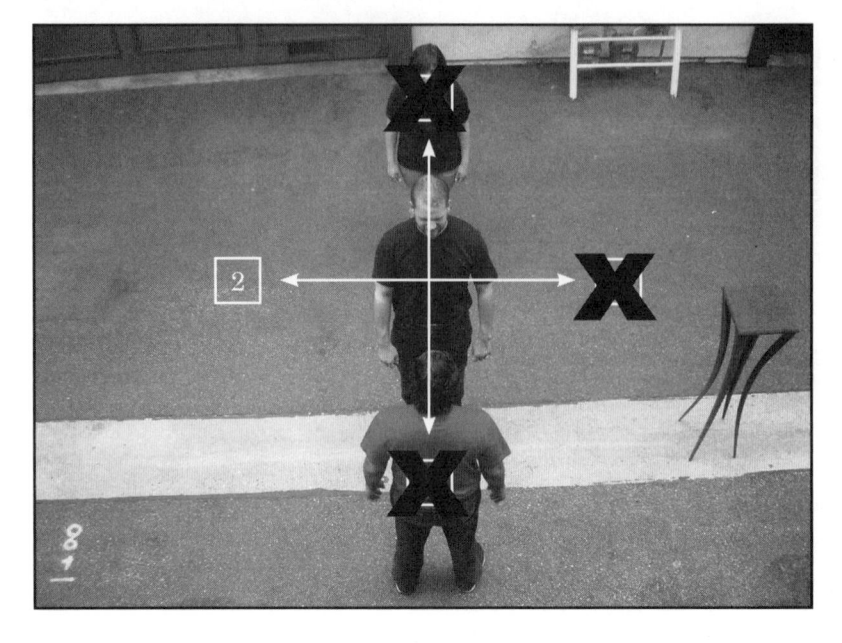

4. Assess which areas are viable and which are not:
    - Diamond 1 - Assailant
    - Diamond 2 - Free
    - Diamond 3 - Obstacle (Person)
    - Diamond 4 - Obstacle (Table)

STRIKE ZONES

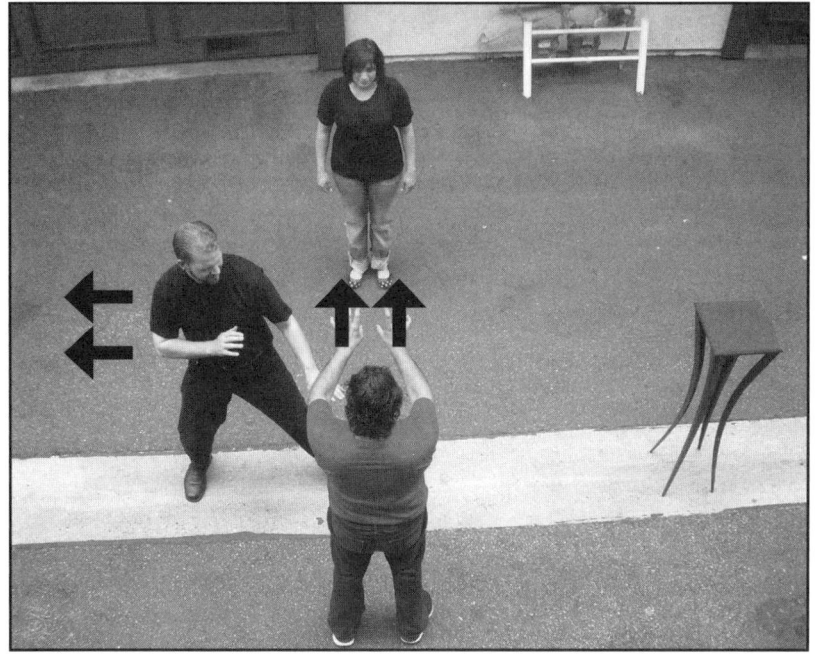

5. QUICKLY MOVE TO DIAMOND POINT 2 (FREE PATH) AS THE ATTACKER STEPS IN.

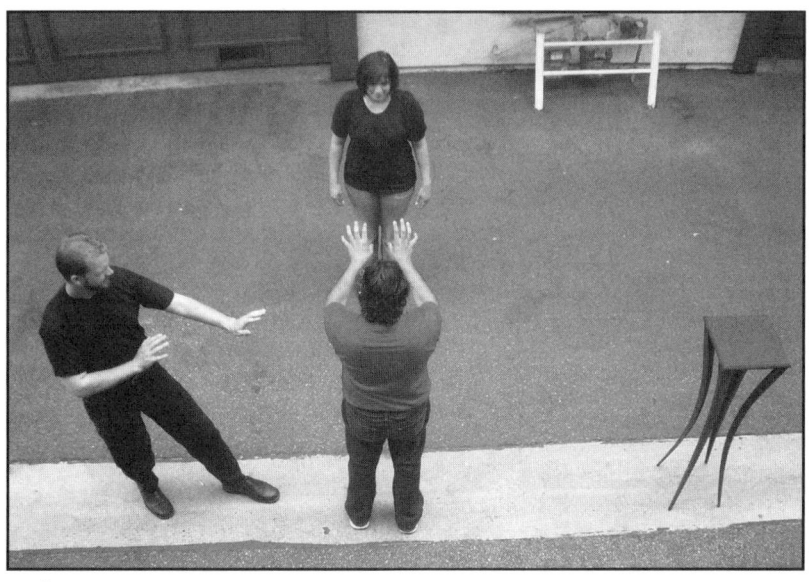

6. ONCE MOVEMENT IS COMPLETE, RESET AND READY FOR CONTINUED ATTACKS.

HAND & ARM ATTACKS

CHAPTER 2
HAND & ARM ATTACKS

In this chapter we learn the proper positioning of several effective offensive and defensive hand techniques, including variations of both closed fist and open hand. With the simple changing of finger position, one's attack can increase in effectiveness tenfold.

Proper hand attacks do come from a finite source, but with the several options listed in this chapter, you will never find yourself without a well chosen method of attack. You may incorporate and interchange your attacks to your own personal liking and comfort. Consider however that your first choice may not always be a possibility. A slight injury, a lack of space, or even your clothing can limit your opportunities. The instructions below prepare you for even the worst-case scenarios. With decades of Kung Fu experience behind me, I have many times appreciated the teaching concept of knowing what to do **when** things go wrong, not *if*. Personally, I have many times had to vary my style of fighting due to surroundings and environment.

Working at "Balboa", a higher-end club on the sunset strip, I had to show restraint, discretion, and stealth. When a customer would step out of line, I would have to use precise strikes, quickly hitting nerve points and quietly removing them from the premises. Most of the time the other customers would have no awareness that the altercation had even happened. Unfortunately, I experienced a darker, flip side to this coin as well.

Upon my first big night as Head of Security for the nightclub, "The Lounge", we on the security team were told by the manager that a new, huge promotion would be coming and that we were expected to "send a message." His meaning was to use a display of force that would dissuade future rowdiness for all of the clubs promotions. The club, until this point, maintained a calm atmosphere and had been easy to control. However, this first large campaign would change all of that. Knowing that the well publicized night would bring

HAND & ARM ATTACKS

hundreds of people together in a cramped area, we borrowed several extra members from one of the club's sister-properties.

Add together alcohol, testosterone, and a ready security team and you have quite a mix. What ensued next was a melee including full contact moshing, aggressors being lifted and thrown backwards down flights of stairs, and an assembly-line like atmosphere of bouncers choking out and removing violent drunks from the premises. The strange consideration in all of this is that though my situation changed dramatically between these two nights, my moves did not need to follow suit. With slight alterations to my existing techniques and positions, I found that I was still able to utilize the skills that were always the most comfortable for me.

As you will see, upper body attacks can easily change from the stealth of a precise pressure point strike to a bold, full fisted punch to your attacker's nose. One thing never alters though; you must maintain control of yourself and your decisions at all times. Consider what techniques are best for every situation, not how good it would feel to open-handedly slap your assailant to the ground. You should consider the following only as options for your success, not guarantees.

Another advantage is also attained with this chapter's lessons. Shifting style makes any opponent difficult to read. Whereas you may only be one fighter, you will constantly be able to shift to many different defenses. Many times I have thrown an opponent off by simply changing my hand position, thus changing my attack. Whether a bouncer in a nightclub or a fighter on the street, this shifting causes intimidation to be as much a factor for effective combat as physical skill is. Having said that, in this chapter we will analyze the positioning for open and willing strikes, quiet submissions through pressure points, and everything else in between.

Punches by definition are considered to be closed hand attacks. While the target of the punch is almost always forward, the origin may not always be so. As true as this is, so is the truth that punches do not need to look similar or traditional. Pictured and described below, the reader will learn to recognize the differences between a fully formed and partially formed fist and all of the necessary variations.

HAND & ARM ATTACKS

IMPORTANT SAFETY INFORMATION

1. When choosing a striking method, remember the rule: **Bone never goes against bone**. If you are hitting a hard surface such as the head, make sure to use a "soft" attack such as a palm strike.

2. Consider that while we focus on the upper body in this chapter, all of the strength in these strikes should originate with the twisting of your hips.

3. When making a fist, be certain to use only the lowest knuckles of your index and middle finger (see below). *Star Fist/Eagles Beak, and knuckle rakes are partial fists and listed and shown as exceptions.*

Proper Striking Area

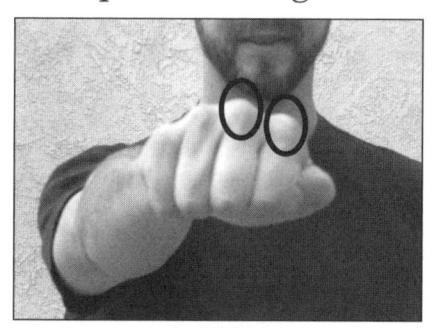

FULL FIST STRIKING AREA

Hand Attacks

Fingers, Palm, Knuckles, Chop, the hand offers a bevy of opportunities to strike at your opponent. With regular practice these options make us nothing less than versatile and effective in even the worst of situations. In the following pages are some of the most useful and efficient positions you can produce during any attack.

Whole Fist

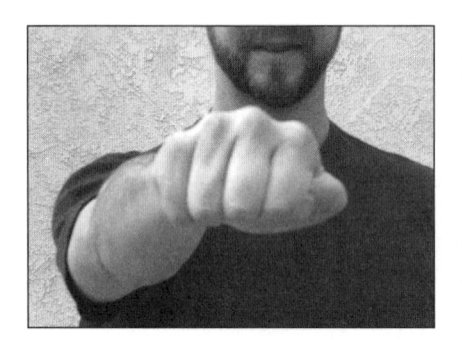

A whole fist is what most consider to be the standard punch. The wrist twists inward toward the thumb during punch until the back of the hand faces upward. The spinning action of the wrist in motion produces a great amount of torque, increasing the punch's effectiveness.

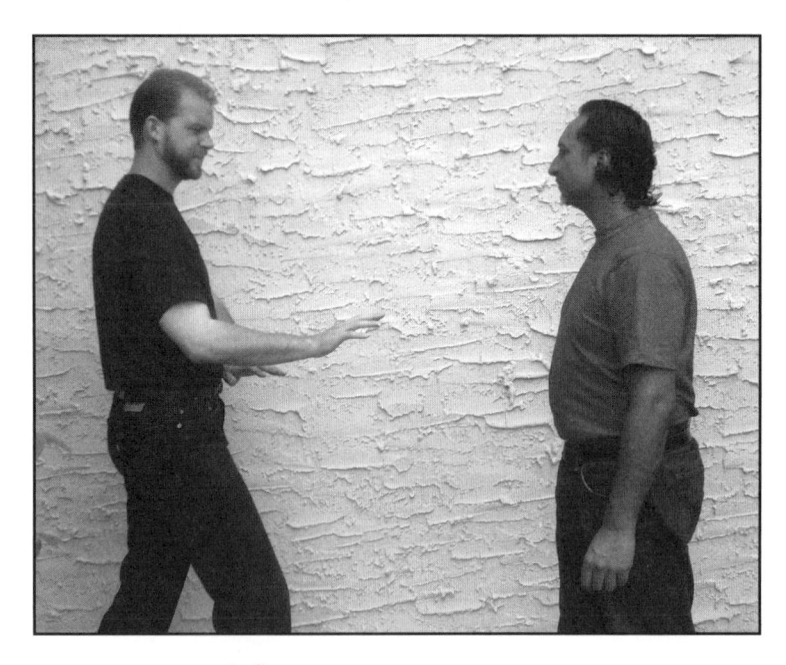

1. STANDING AT READY POSITION.

HAND & ARM ATTACKS

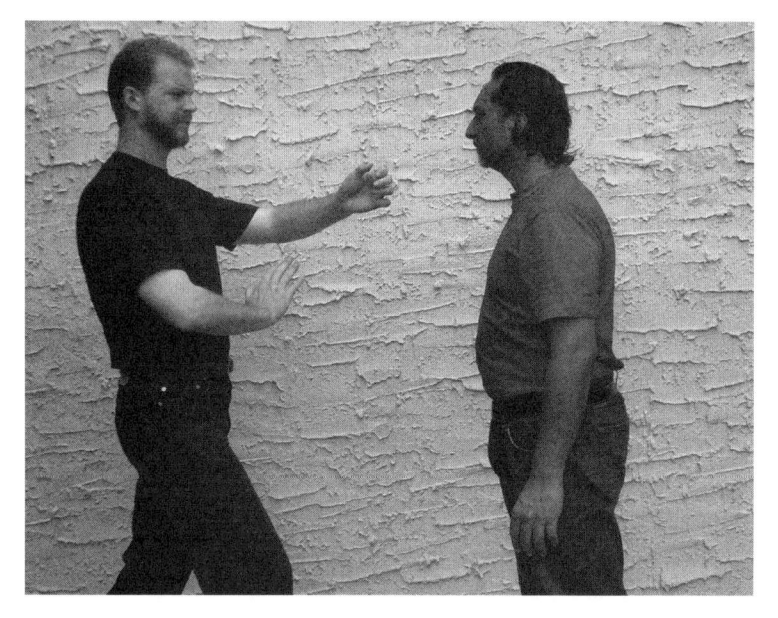

2. Move your hand forward, twisting inward toward the thumb.

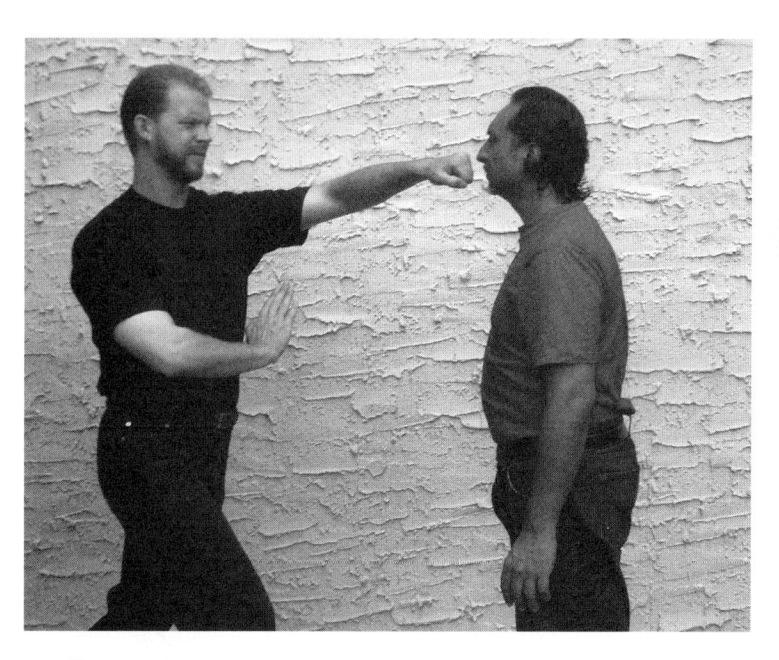

3. Complete the punch with the back of hand facing upward.

HAND & ARM ATTACKS

Half Fist

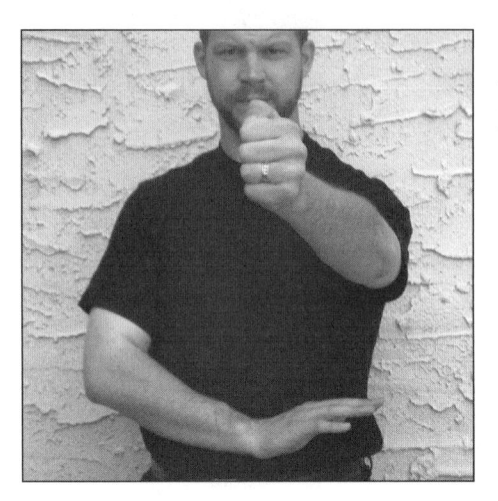

A half fist is achieved by closing the hand as usual, but utilizing a half twist and leaving the thumb pressed securely on top of the hand. While this will not administer the same amount of torque and pressure of a "Whole Fist" punch, it is considered by many experts as a superior attack due to the elbow's ability to quickly protect the midsection.

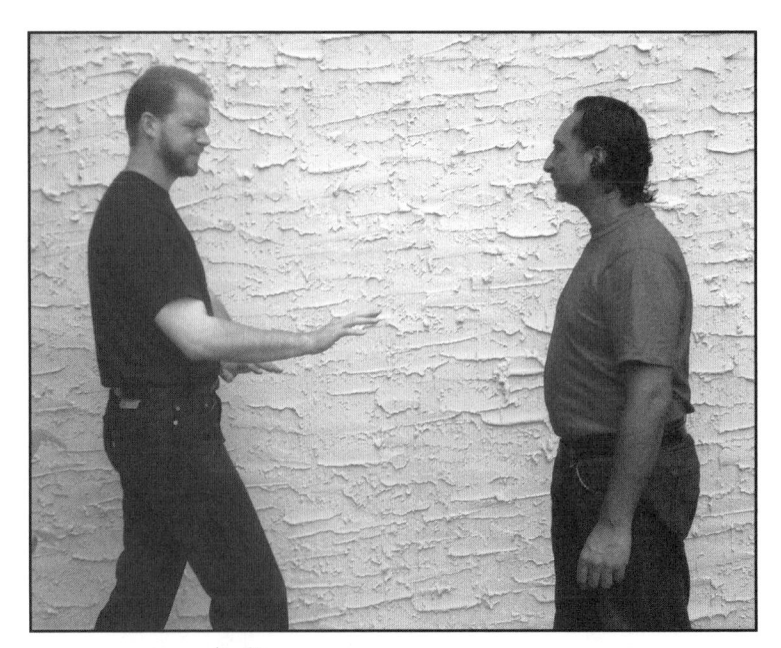

1. STANDING AT READY POSITION.

HAND & ARM ATTACKS

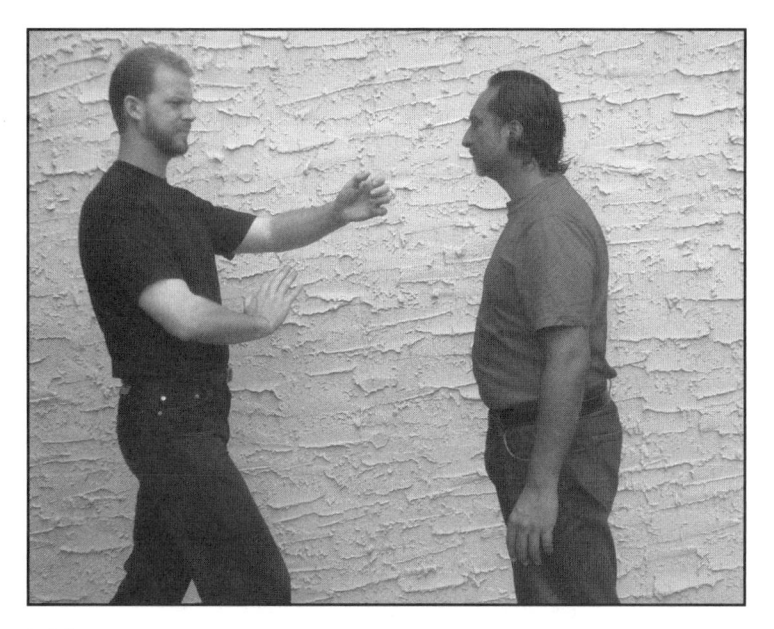

2. Move your hand forward, twisting inward toward the thumb.

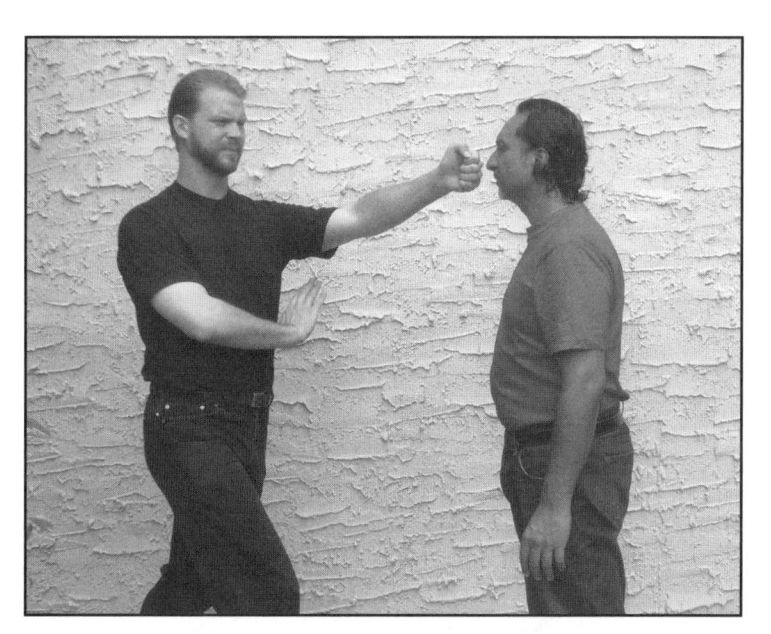

3. Complete the punch with thumb facing upward.

Backfist

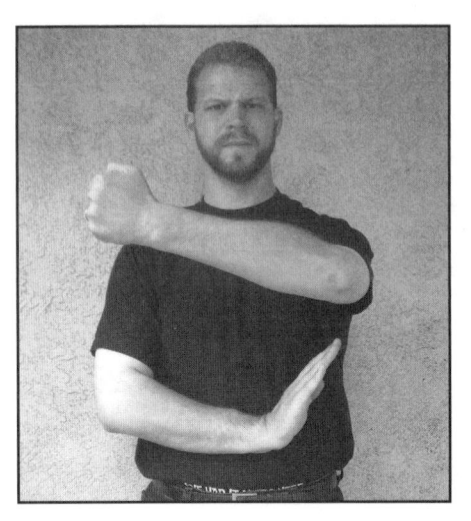

With the same hand position of a Half Fist, the Backfist provides its powerful attack from an outside swinging motion. The same rules apply as did with Whole and Half Fists, only the bottom knuckles of the index and middle fingers may be used.

Using a standard punch, a backfist is achieved by swinging the closed hand in an arc motion to the desired target. Even though attack is of a different angle, make sure only to use the index and middle finger knuckles and not the back of the hand.

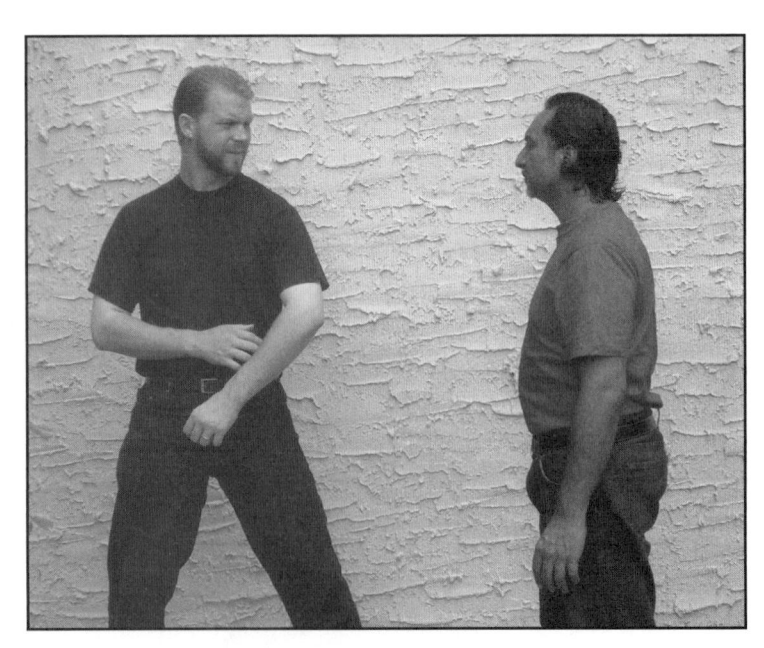

1. STANDING AT READY POSITION.

HAND & ARM ATTACKS

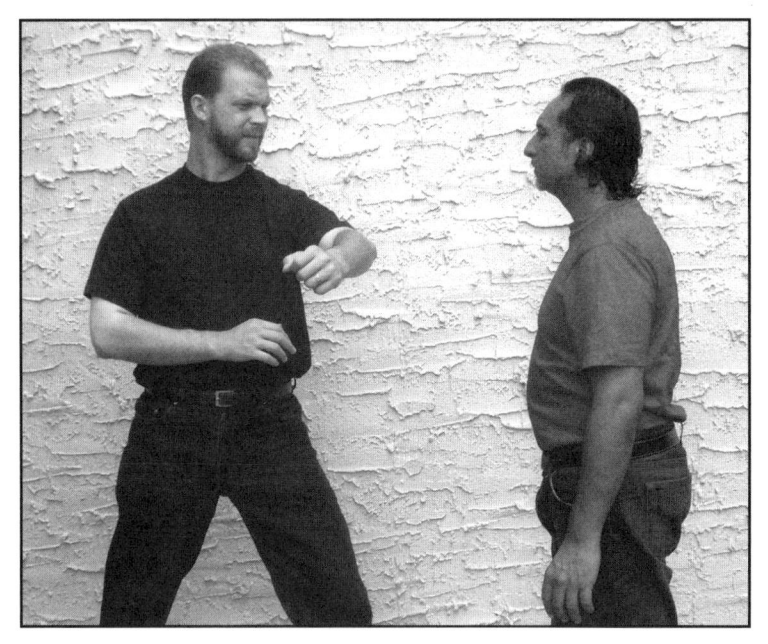

2. Move your front hand inward using a swinging motion toward opponent.

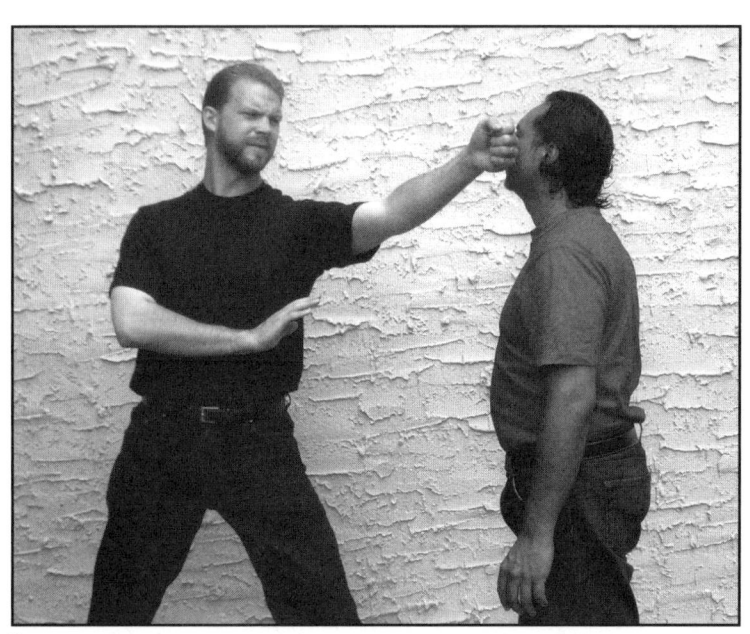

3. Complete the punch by landing the top two knuckles against opponent.

Knuckle Fist

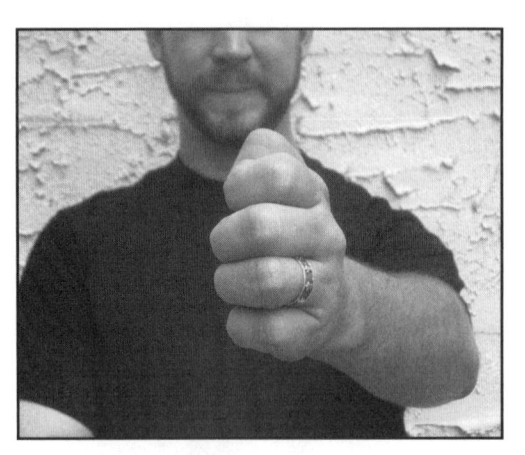

Allowing for a sharper, elongated attack, Knuckle fists and rakes are punches made by partially opening a half fist, but keeping the fingers bent to expose the middle knuckles. Both Knuckle Fists and Rakes allow for greater reach and a sharper more pin-pointed strike. The position for both strikes is identical, however the attacks are quite different.

Knuckle Fists are used with a straight forward motion, whereas Knuckle Rakes are swung in from the side in a circular movement.

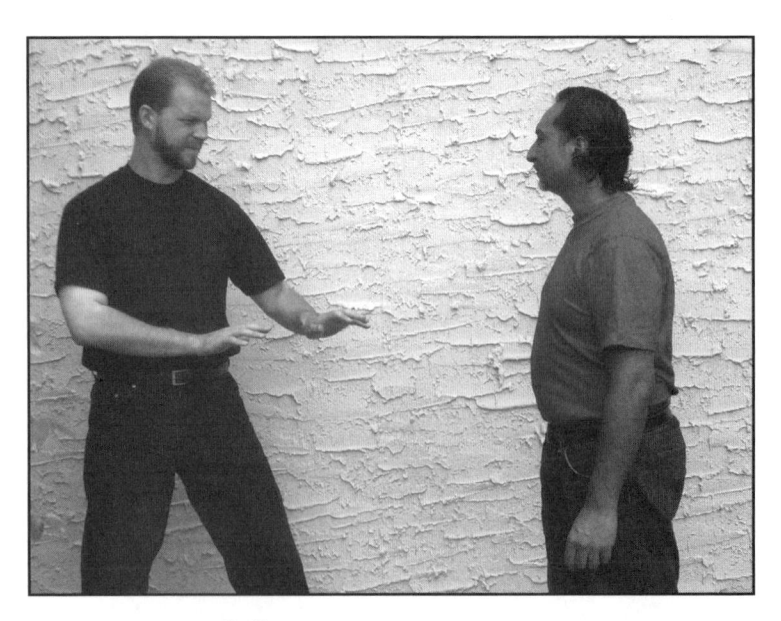

1. STANDING AT READY POSITION.

HAND & ARM ATTACKS

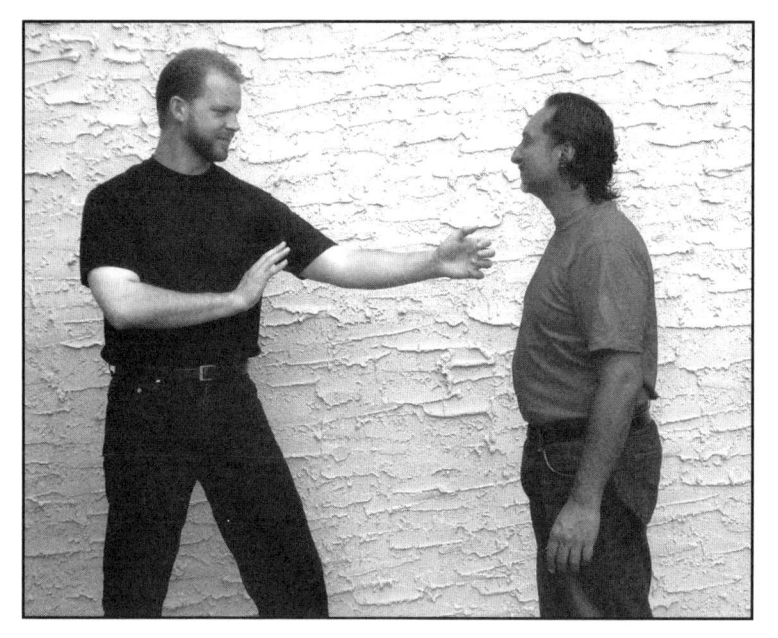

2. Move your striking hand inward toward opponent's chest.

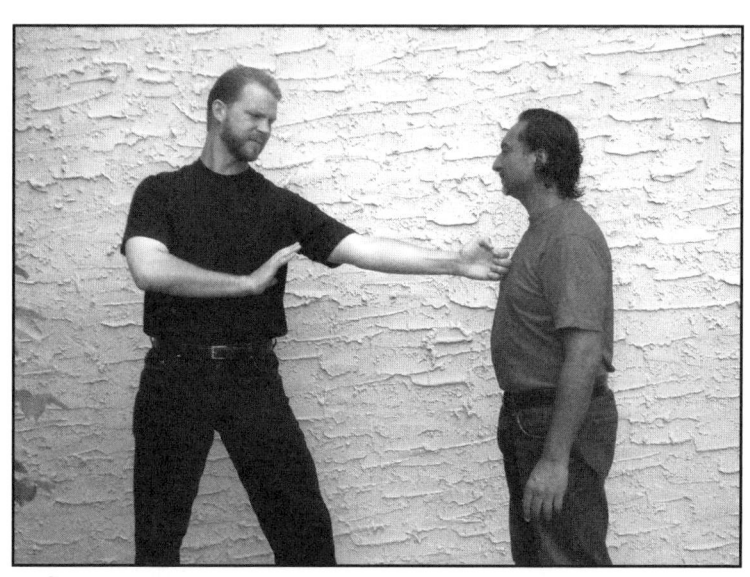

3. Complete the punch by striking the center of opponent's chest with the middle knuckles of your hand.

Star Fist/Eagle's Beak

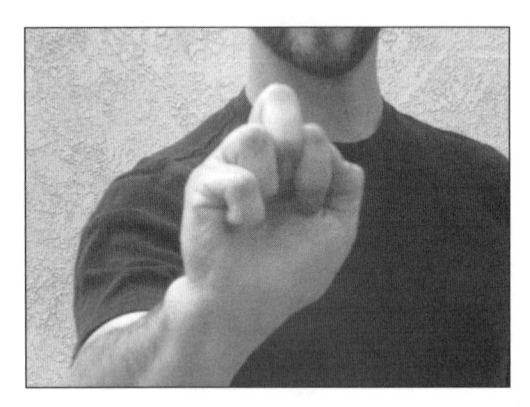

The pressure point variation of a Knuckle Fist, the Star Fist/Eagle's Beak administration is identical excepting the fact that it focuses the entirety of its assault upon the middle knuckle of the middle finger. This attack is perfect for pressure point punches (ex. the temple or sternum).

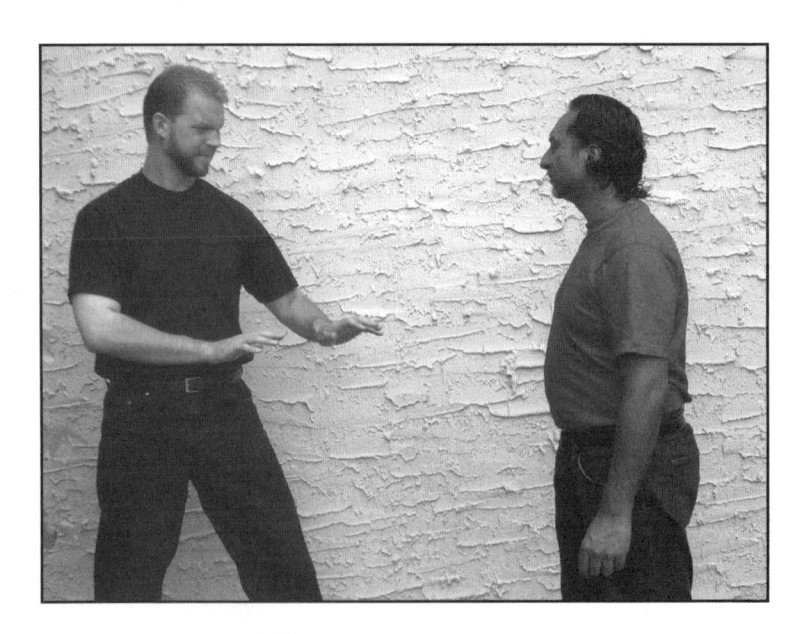

1. STANDING AT READY POSITION.

HAND & ARM ATTACKS

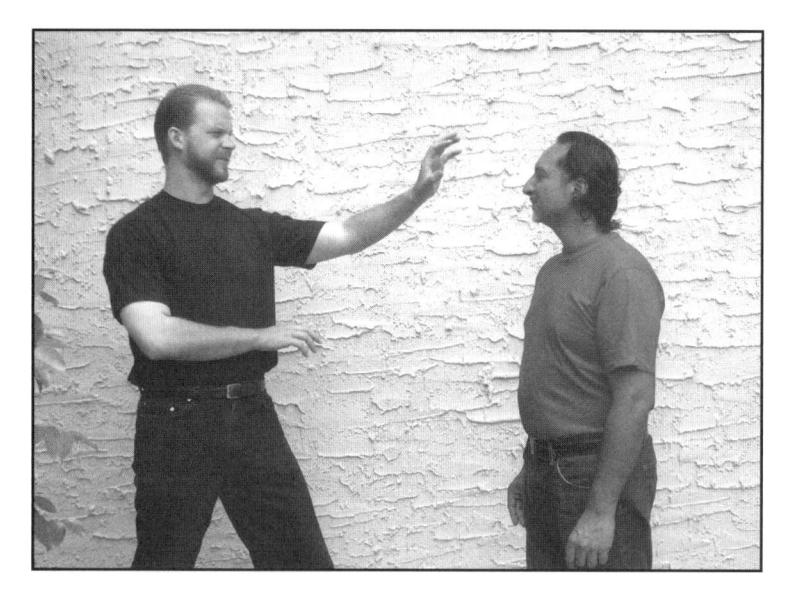

2. Raise your hand upward at opponent's face.

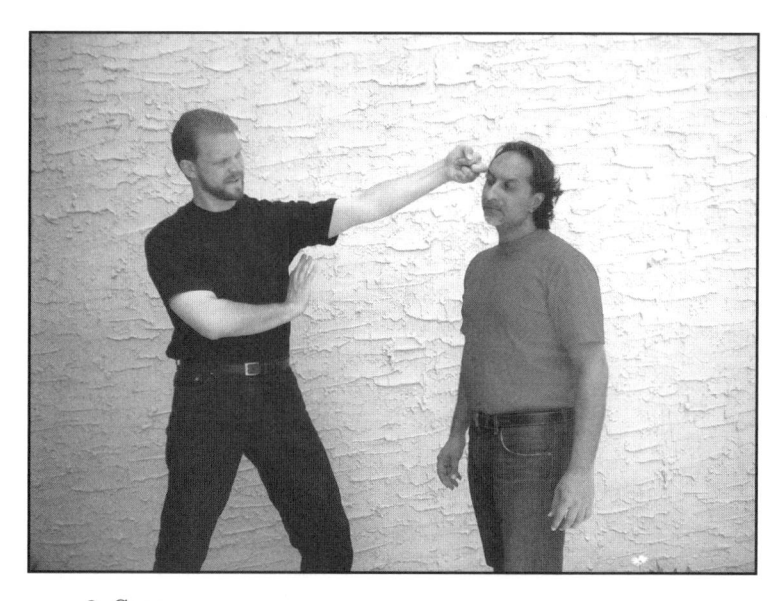

3. Close your fist, leaving the center knuckle extended to strike at opponent's temple.

Finger Gouge

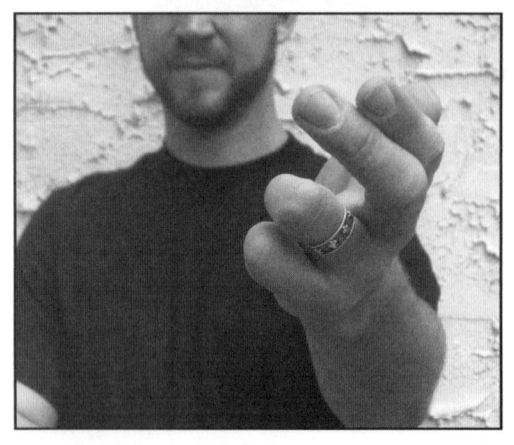

This hit deserves special mention. Too many times it has served me without fail. During one unfortunate evening at the club "The Gate" I found myself running to the V.I.P. section of the club upon an emergency security call. One of the largest men I have ever seen was wildly throwing punches to every person in his vicinity. Steroids make already violent men all the more dangerous. Even at 6'3" and 200 lbs., I knew that I could never match the physical strength of this adversary and I had no desire to even try. My years of training had impressed upon me a vital piece of knowledge. You can't build up muscle over your eye. With one well placed strike, the assailant hit the floor. The point of this recollection is that utility in martial arts is only as difficult as you want it to be. A simple poke can level even the most powerful adversary. For this reason and this reason alone, the eye gouge is included here.

For maximum effectiveness, the middle and index finger are used to attack. Using both fingers ensures proper support of the strike, lessening risk of injury. Make sure that there is a slight bend in all knuckles prior to the strike. After having fully extended the middle and index finger, curl the ring and fourth finger inward towards the palm.

HAND & ARM ATTACKS

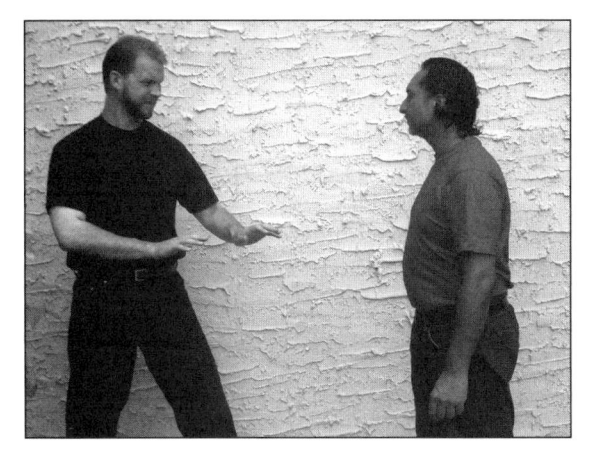

1. STANDING AT READY POSITION.

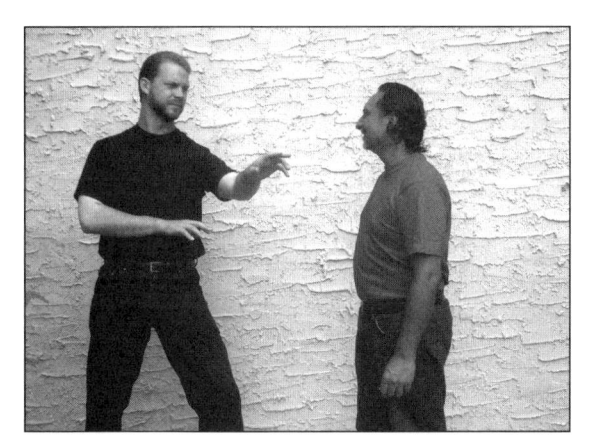

2. RAISE YOUR FRONT HAND, EXTENDING ONLY THE INDEX AND MIDDLE FINGERS.

MAKE CERTAIN TO LEAVE A SLIGHT CURVE IN THE FINGER KNUCKLES.

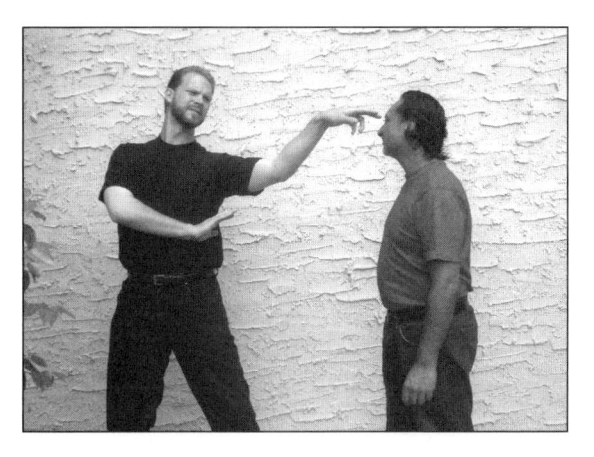

3. COMPLETE THE ATTACK BY STRIKING YOUR FINGERS INTO OPPONENT'S EYE.

HAND & ARM ATTACKS

Thumb Spike

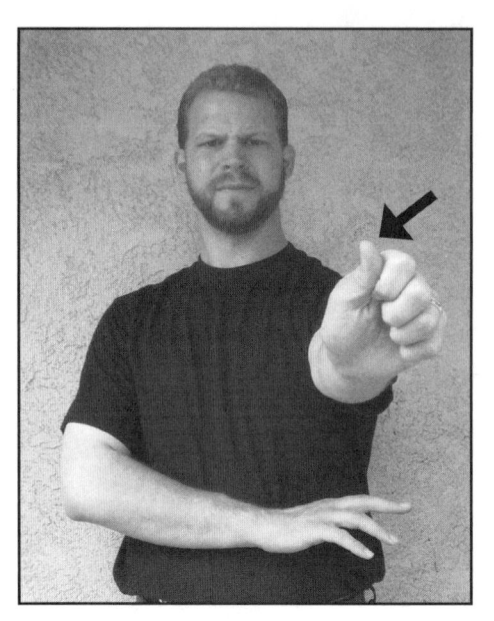

Proper positioning for a pressure point strike can be easily achieved by establishing a thumb spike. After forming a knuckle fist, slightly extend the thumb over the index finger. Due to the angle of the bone at the top of the thumb, you can strike an opponent with adequate force without concerning yourself with personal injury. Squeezing the pad of the thumb against the inside of the index finger's middle knuckle, hold your fist closed and braced for pressure point impact.

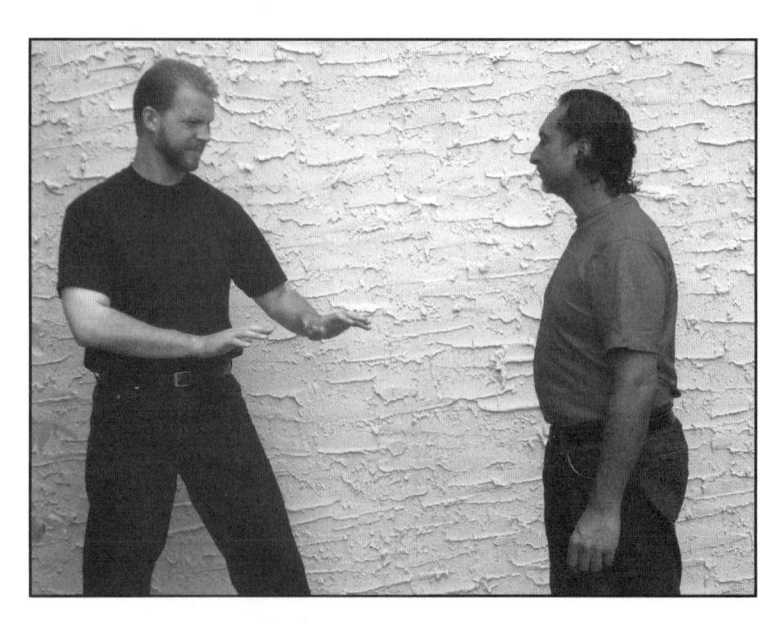

1. STANDING AT READY POSITION.

HAND & ARM ATTACKS

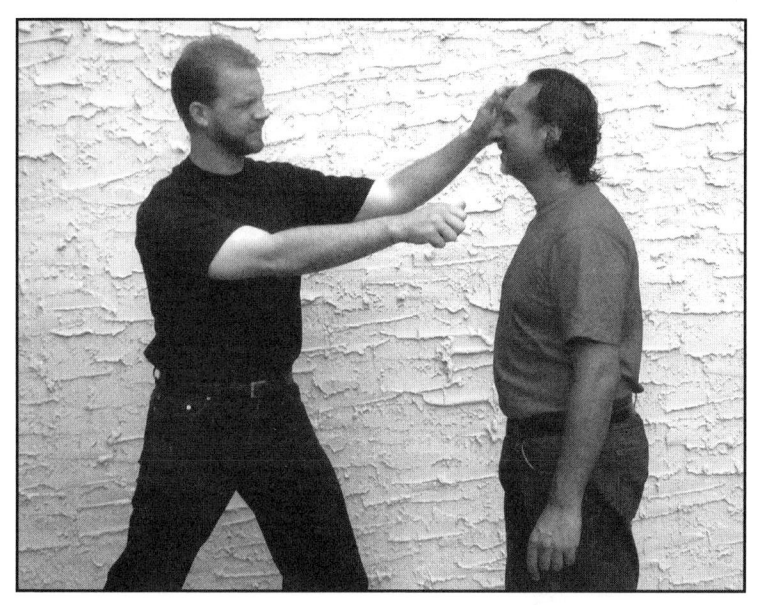

2. Move both hands forward, using one to grab at the side of the opponent's head while the other closes into a fist with an extended thumb tip.

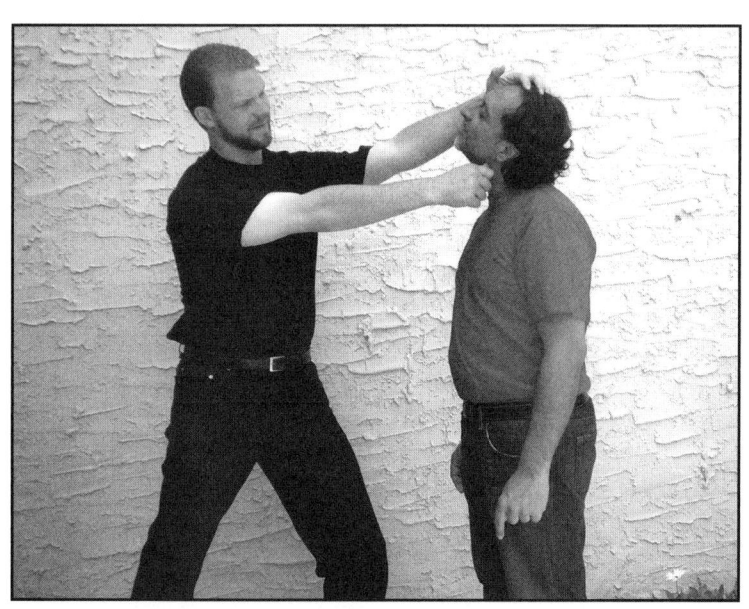

3. Finish the attack by pressing the tip of the thumb firmly directly behind the opponent's ear lobe and providing supporting pressure with the other hand.

HAND & ARM ATTACKS

Palm Strike

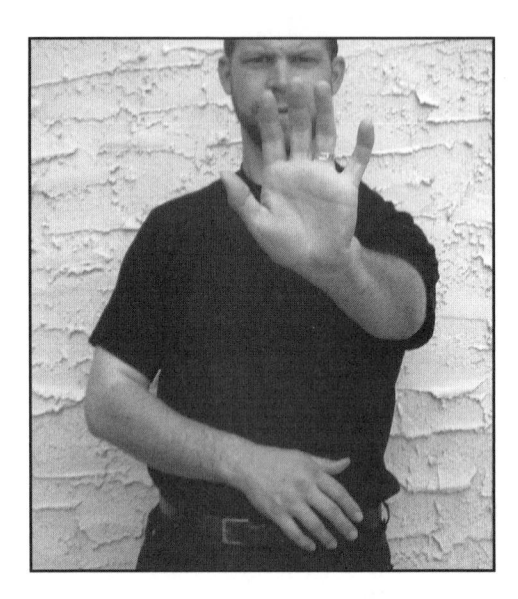

A safe manner of striking no matter what zone you wish to attack, palm strikes are achieved by pressing the outer rim of the palm forward until contact is made with the opponent's body in a forward motion. This attack is perfect for heart strikes.

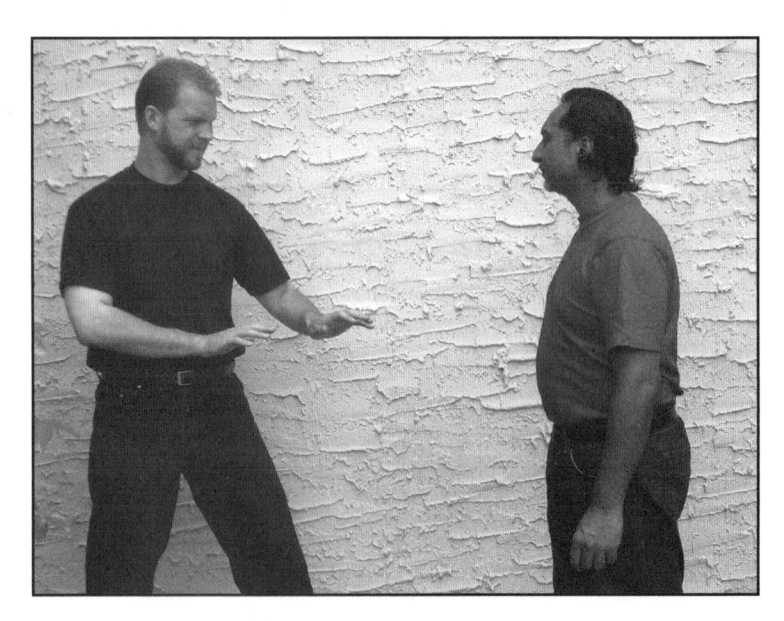

1. STANDING AT READY POSITION.

HAND & ARM ATTACKS

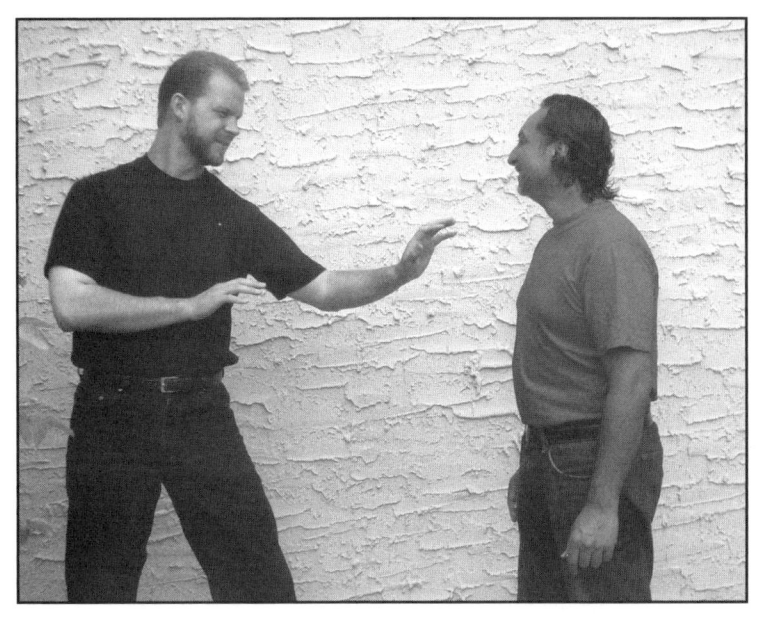

2. Move your hand forward, extending the heel of the palm toward the attacker's chest.

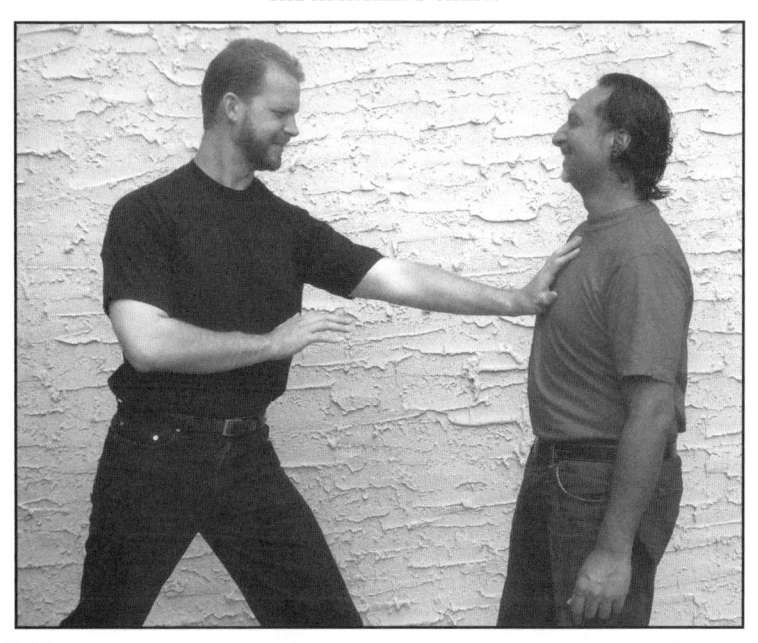

3. Finish the attack by striking your palm over the opponent's heart.

HAND & ARM ATTACKS

Claw

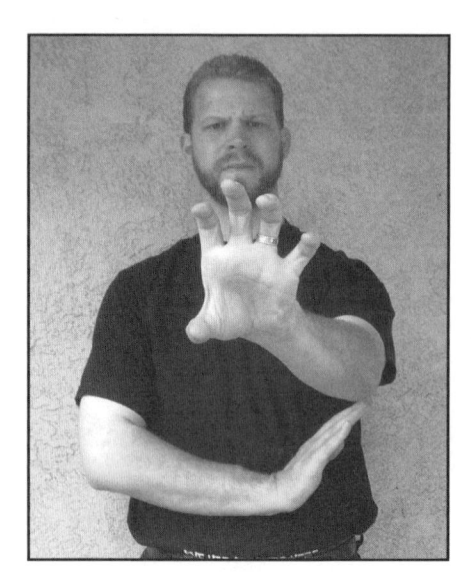

The structure of a claw strike is almost identical with a palm strike, however instead of straightforward attacks, the claw swings in and scratches while delivering a palm strike at the same time. This attack is mostly useful on softer tissue areas of the body (ex. face, back, stomach, etc.)

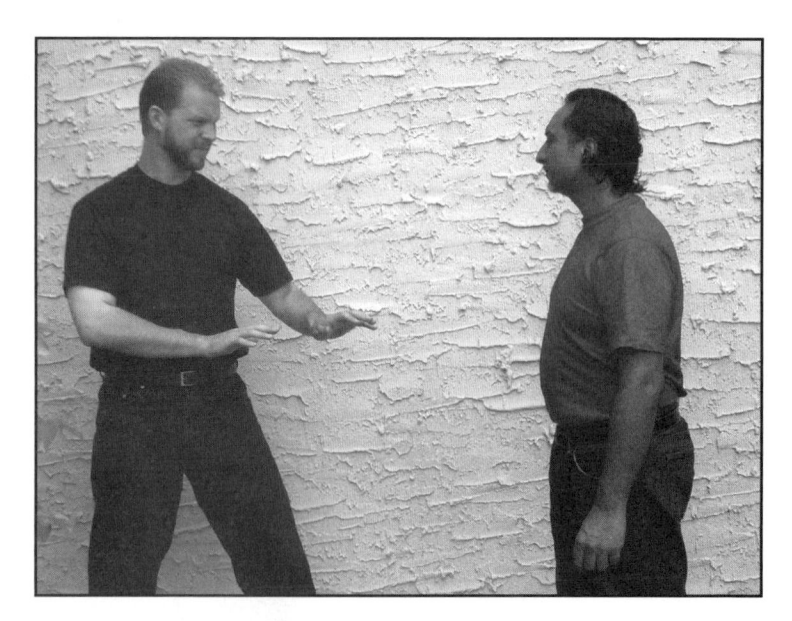

1. STANDING AT READY POSITION.

HAND & ARM ATTACKS

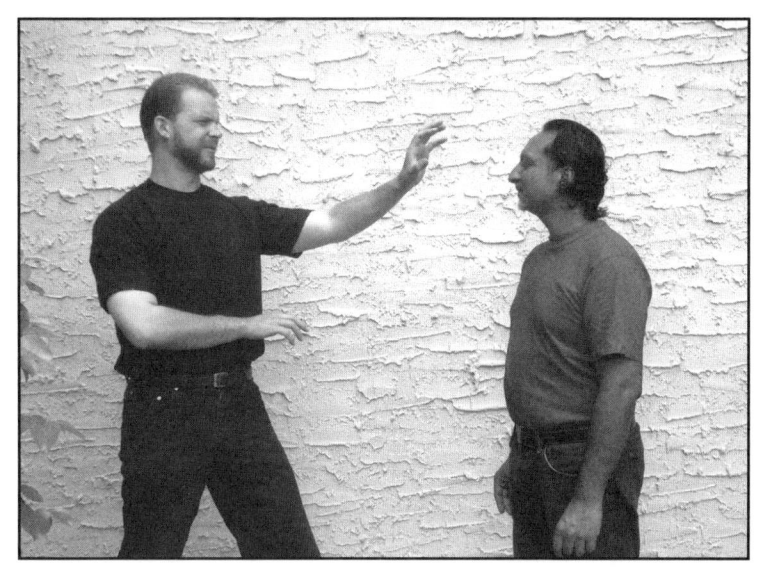

2. Lift your hand upward, opening the palm toward the opponent's face and curling the fingers inward.

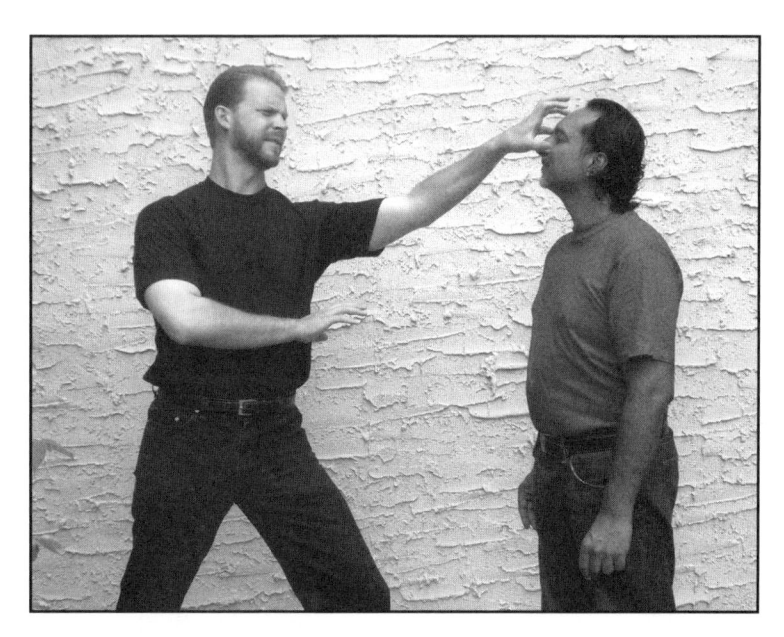

3. Complete the strike by forcing your hand downward, scratching at the opponent's face.

Whip Hand Attack

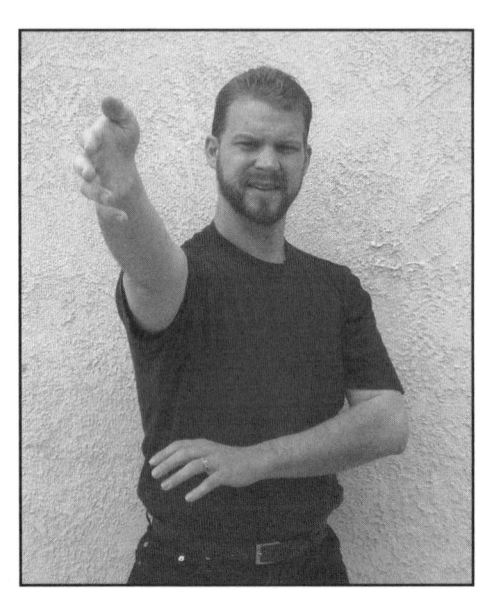

As stated earlier in this chapter, all of your power comes from your hips. Not only is the whip hand the ultimate slap, but it has many times served as the ultimate intimidator. Consider this attack's motion to be akin to throwing a baseball properly. The power comes from your hips, but the swinging action centers around your elbow and works up your arm until "cracking" at your fingertips.

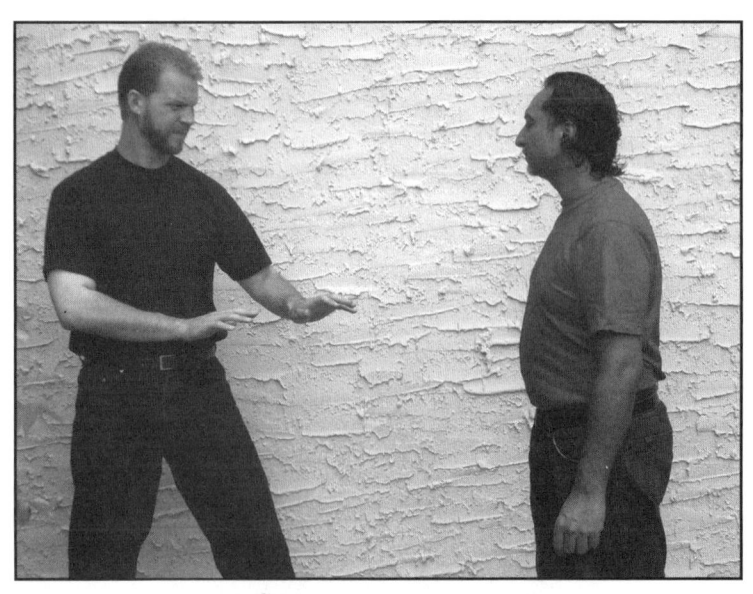

1. STANDING AT READY POSITION.

HAND & ARM ATTACKS

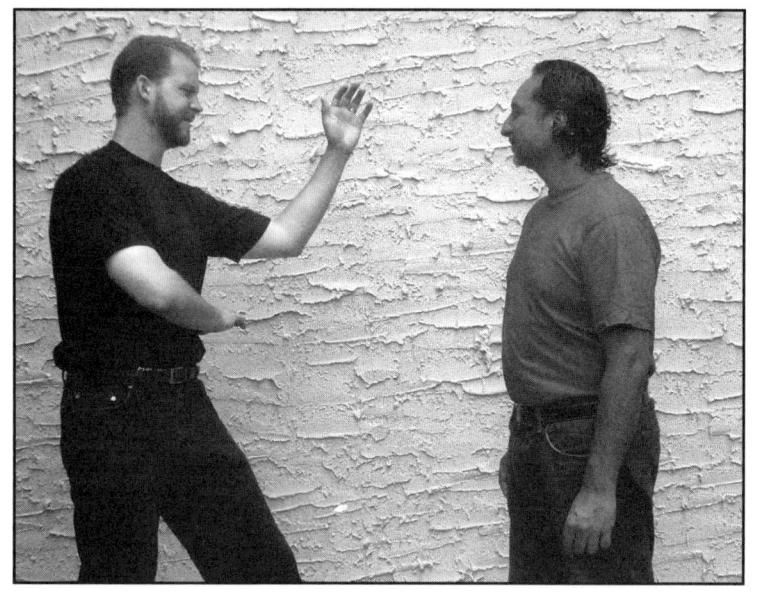

2. Lift your hand upward, twisting the wrist outward and opening the palm.

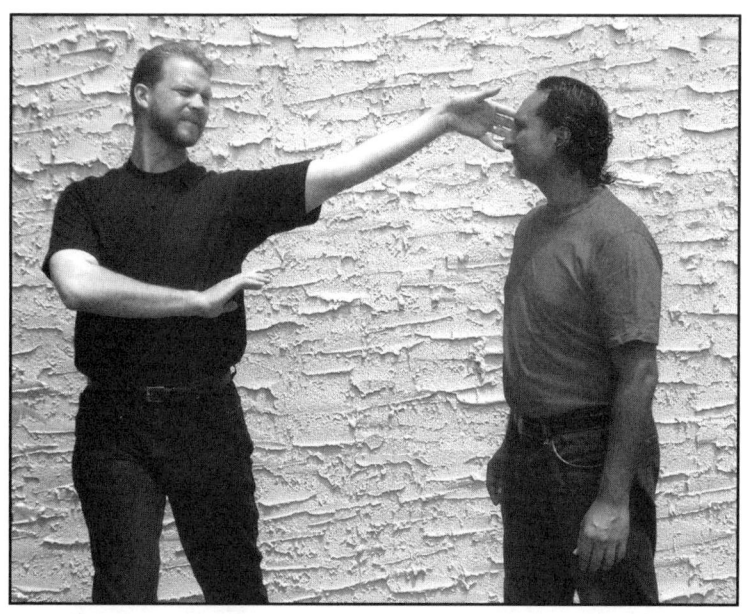

3. Complete the attack by swiftly twisting your hips and striking your fingertips against the opponent's face.

HAND & ARM ATTACKS

Knife Hand

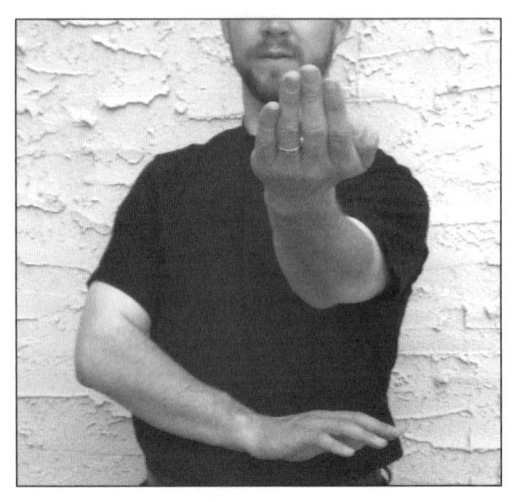

A knife hand allows for the furthest possible reach while maintaining full support of all the fingers striking. *Once again always keep a slight bend in any attacking joints to ensure your safety.* Use a forward thrusting motion unless you wish to use a Chop.

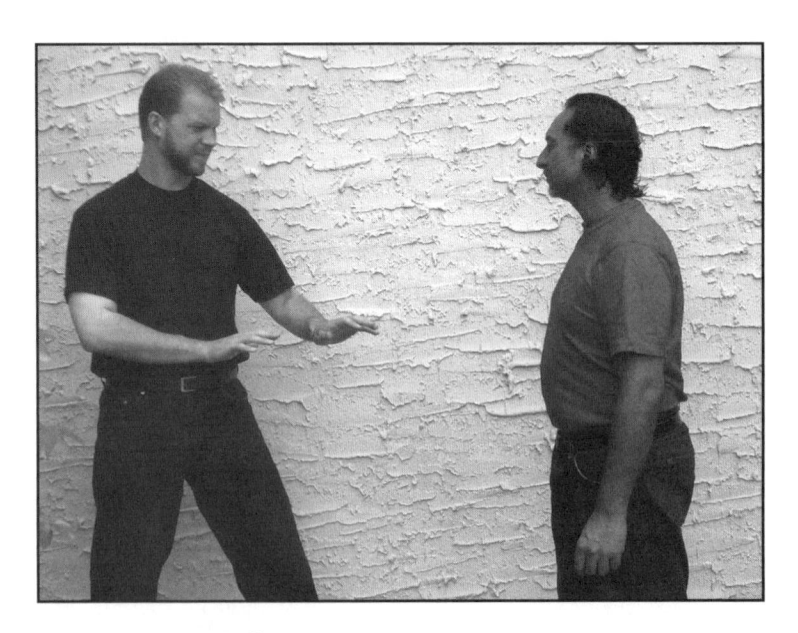

1. STANDING AT READY POSITION.

HAND & ARM ATTACKS

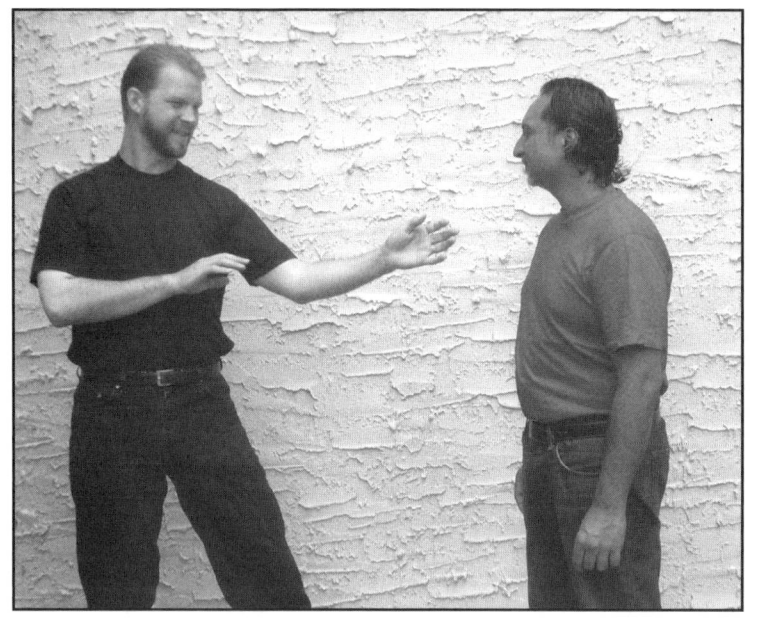

2. BEGIN TO EXTEND YOUR STRIKING HAND, SPINNING THE PALM TO FACE UPWARD.

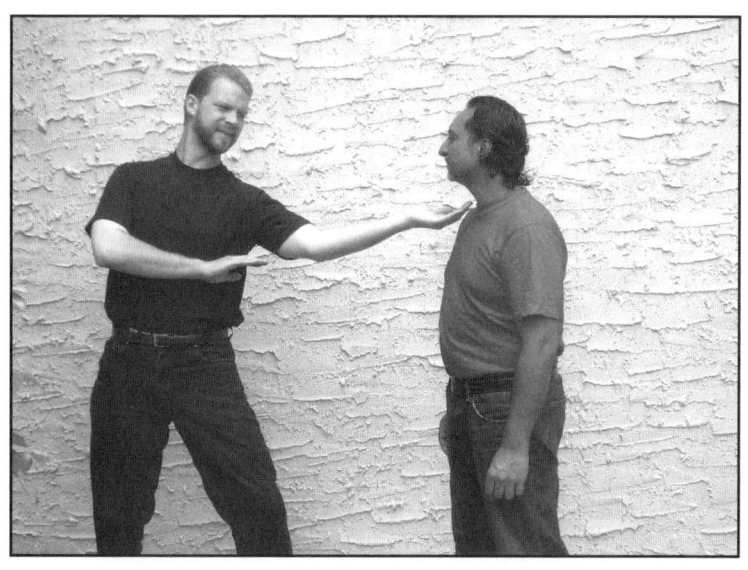

3. COMPLETE THE STRIKE BY FORCING YOUR EXTENDED FINGERTIPS TOWARD OPPONENT'S THROAT. MAKE CERTAIN TO LEAVE A SLIGHT CURVE IN THE FINGER JOINTS.

HAND & ARM ATTACKS

Chop

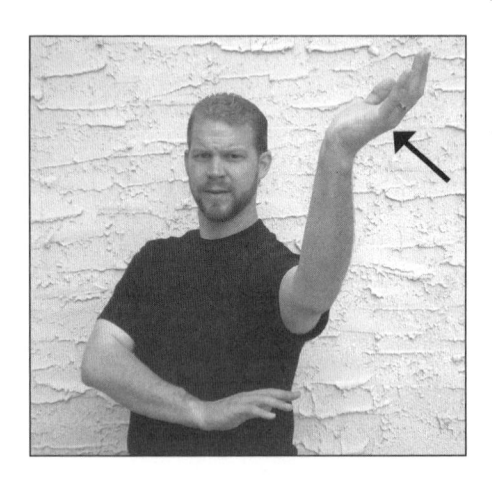

A chop uses the exact same position of a knife hand, but uses an arching motion to administer an attack from the underside of the hand.

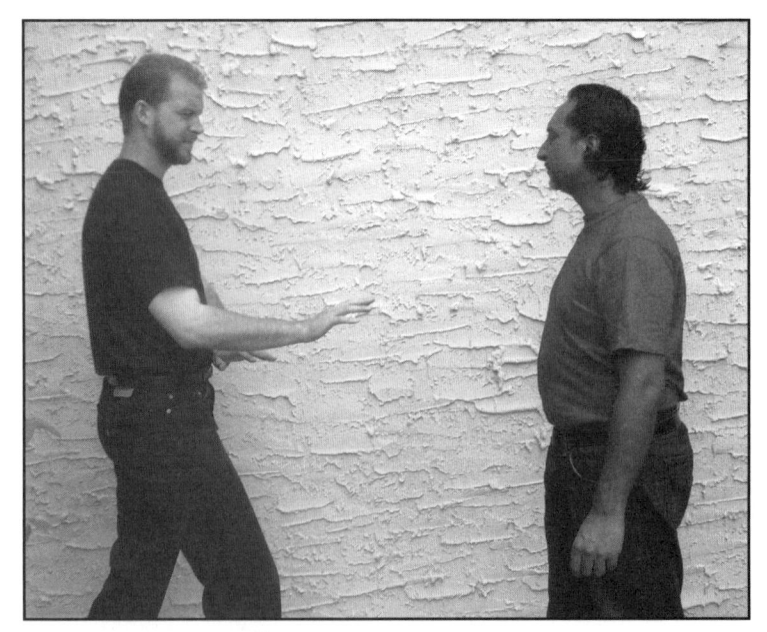

1. STANDING AT READY POSITION.

46

HAND & ARM ATTACKS

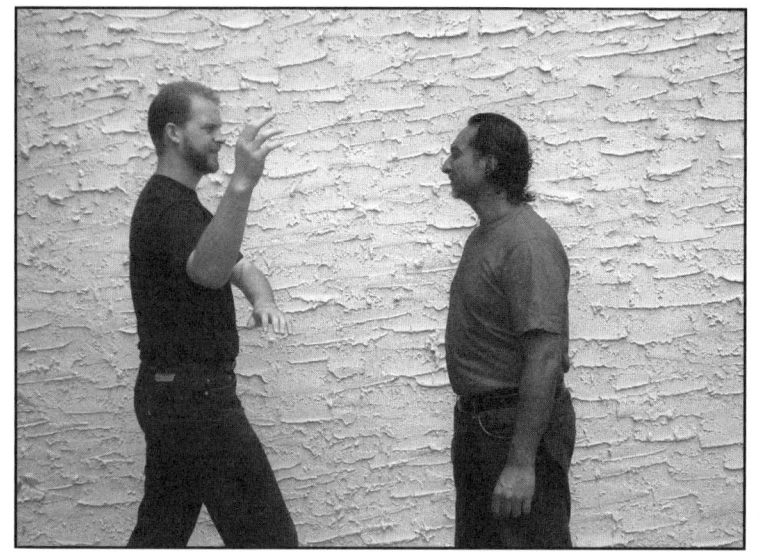

2. Lift your striking hand upward.

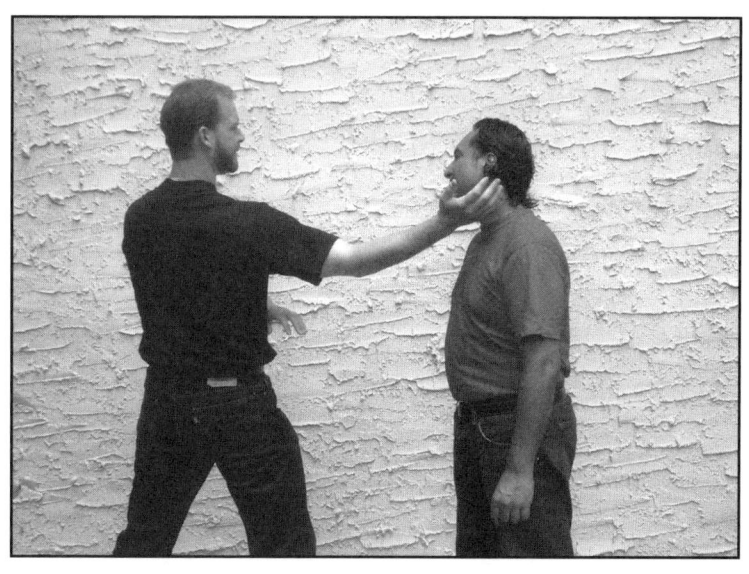

3. Complete the attack by striking the underside of your hand on the opponent's neck.

Arm Attacks

For close quarter attacks in which palm strikes and whip hands are not a possibility, such as strikes made to the side of your opponent's head, wrist and forearm strikes may achieve the desired defense. Make sure to use ONLY the underside and top of the forearm and wrist, not the sides. This will prevent breaking or bruising of bones and joints. Swing your arm inward toward the desired target. *Note: Due to the lack of exposed bone, the forearm and wrist strike attacks are considered to be soft attacks. They may be used against any hard surface of an assailant.*

Wrist Strike

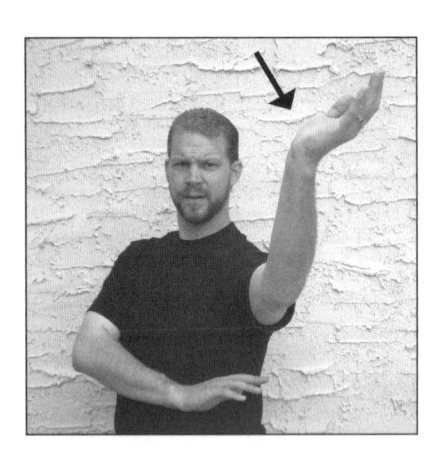

When open-handed attacks are not appropriate due to their lack of blunt force, wrist strikes are more than capable of landing forcefully to the side of your opponent's head.

HAND & ARM ATTACKS

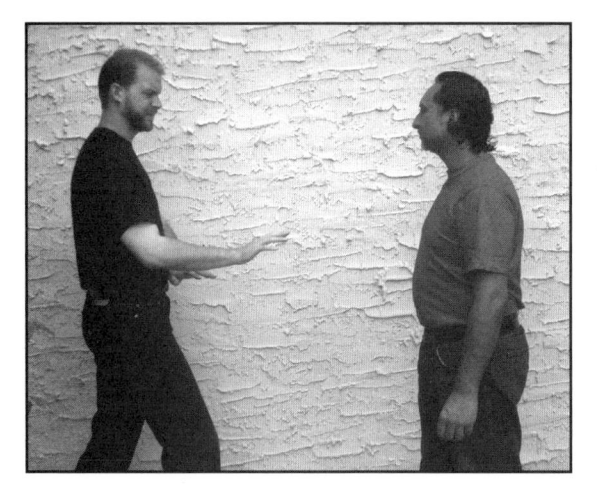

1. STANDING AT READY POSITION.

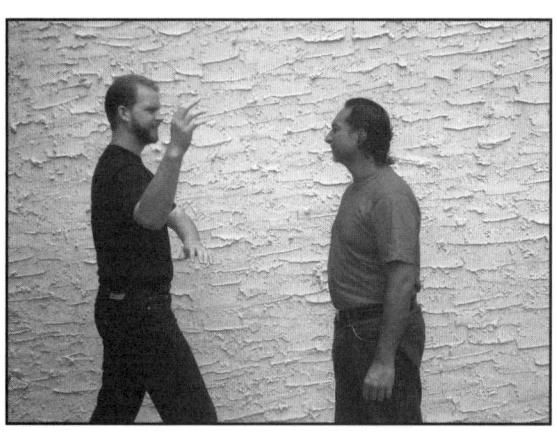

2. LIFT YOUR STRIKING HAND UPWARD AND READY IT TO SWING FORCEFULLY INWARD.

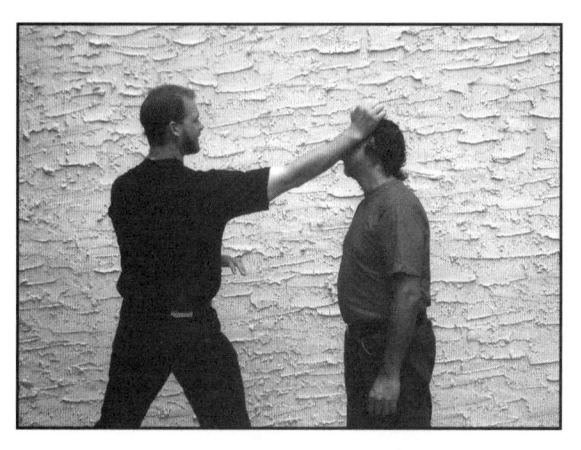

3. COMPLETE THE STRIKE BY LANDING THE INSIDE OF YOUR WRIST AGAINST THE SIDE OF THE OPPONENT'S FACE.

Forearm Strike

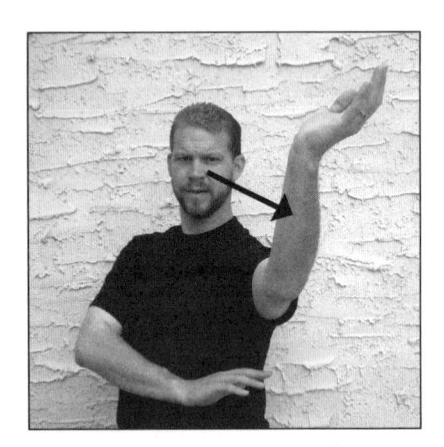

Just as a wrist strike is perfect for blunt force to the head in an extended attack, forearm strikes allow for the same forceful strike in closer combat situations.

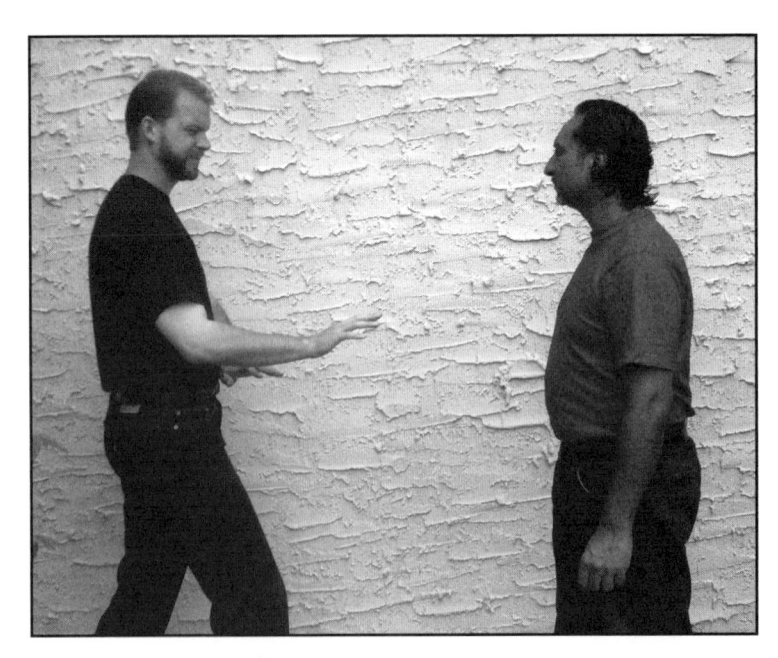

1. STANDING AT READY POSITION.

HAND & ARM ATTACKS

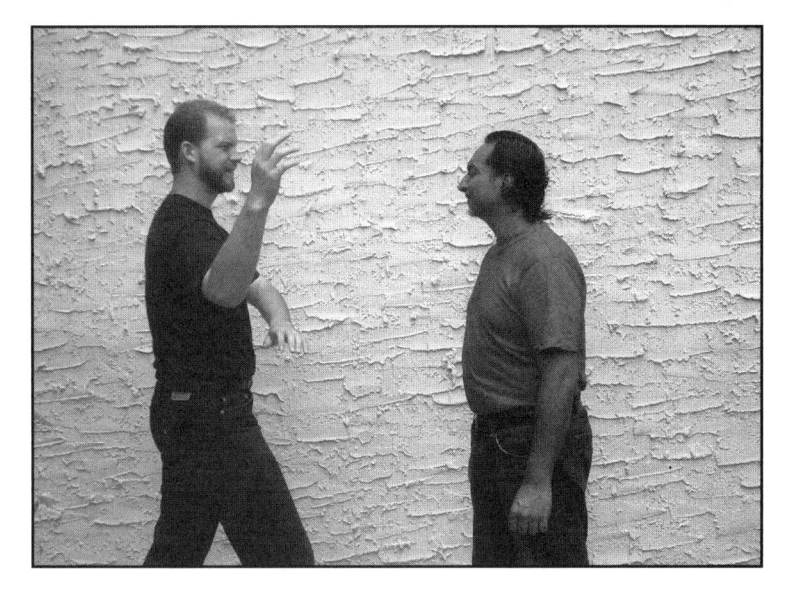

2. Lift your striking hand upward and ready it to swing forcefully inward.

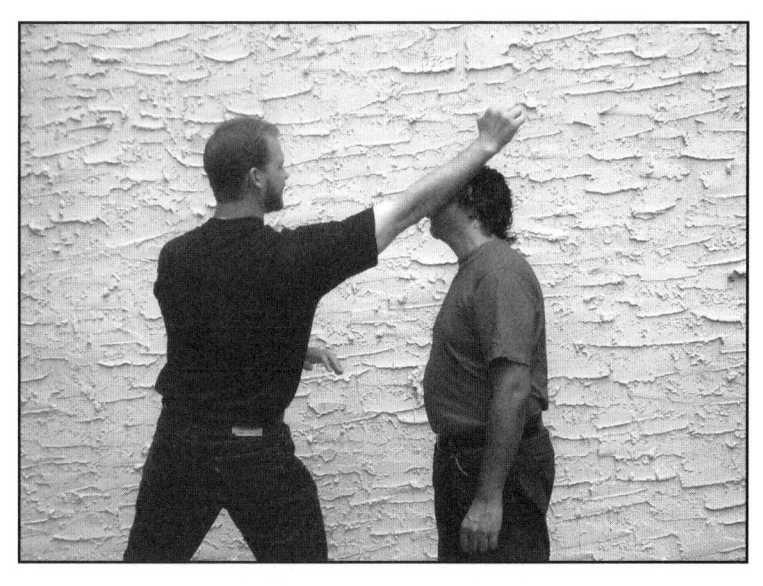

3. Complete the strike by landing the inside of your forearm against the side of the opponent's face.

Elbow Strikes

These strikes offer both forceful brush-by attacks and devastating arcing swings. Consider that proper usage of either strike comes as if a punch was attempted, failed and the elbow happened as an after effect. For proper application, remember to use the tip of your elbow.

Important Note: Make certain to guard your ribcage with your free hand during the application of any elbow strike. Unintentional strikes often occur from attacker's while they are falling.

Obtuse Elbow Strike

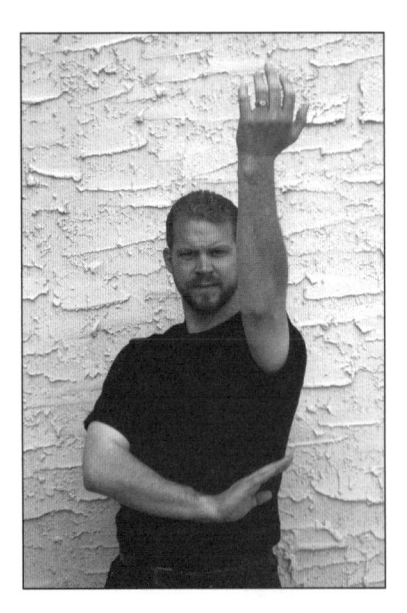

Obtuse Elbow Strikes allow for the continuance of forward motion while teaming with the hard surface of your elbow. Many is the time when a missed opportunity (your punch) can be regained by an obtuse elbow strike.

HAND & ARM ATTACKS

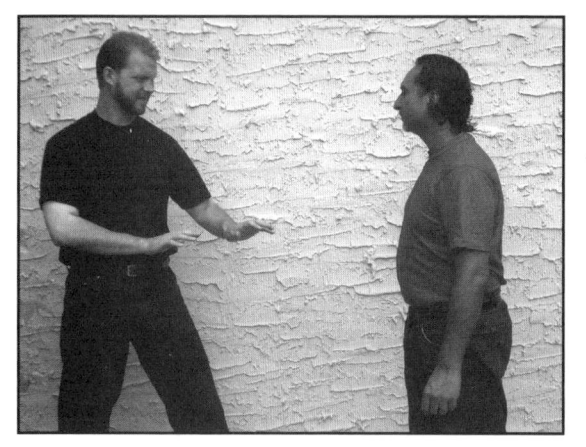

1. STANDING AT READY POSITION.

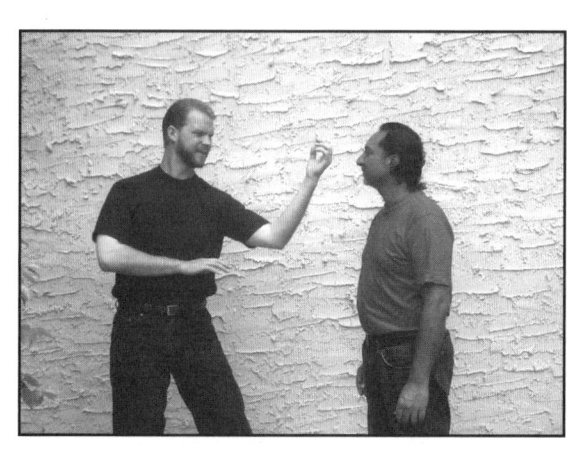

2. RAISE YOUR ARM UPWARD, EXTENDING THE ELBOW FORWARD.

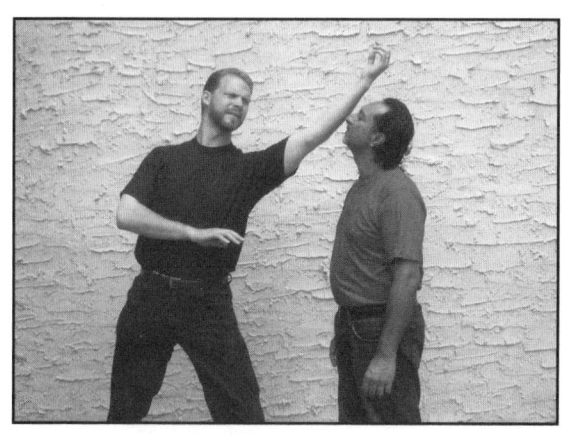

3. COMPLETE THE ATTACK BY "PUNCHING" OVER THE OPPONENT'S HEAD AND LANDING YOUR ELBOW ON THE FACE.

HAND & ARM ATTACKS

Acute Elbow Strike

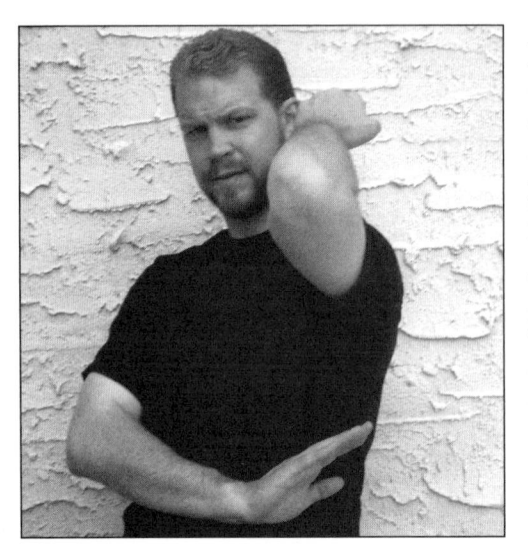

Destruction, destruction, destruction. An acute angle elbow strike is amazingly similar to swinging a ball-pein hammer at someone. It has a massive force lent behind it and a sharp tip that will penetrate even the fattiest part of the human body. It can be used by itself or used to crush with the assistance of your free hand, such as in a 4 point destruction rolling fist. (See Chapter 3)

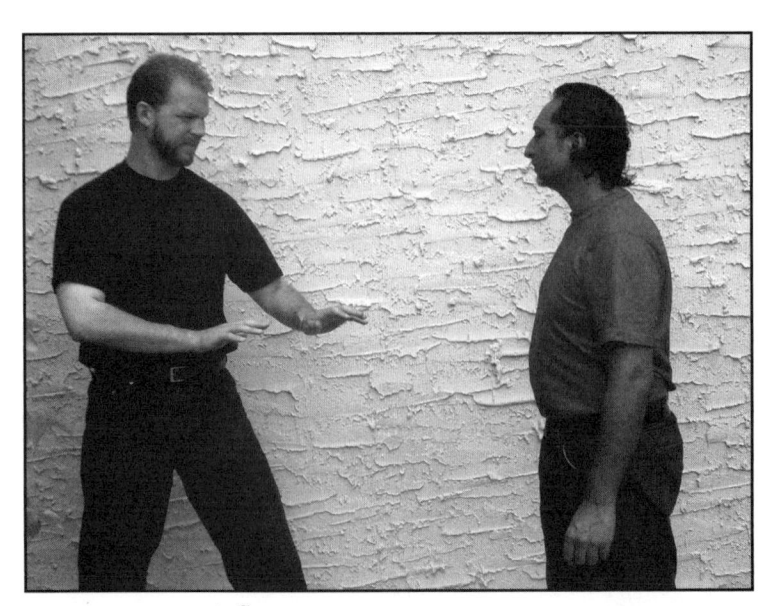

1. STANDING AT READY POSITION.

HAND & ARM ATTACKS

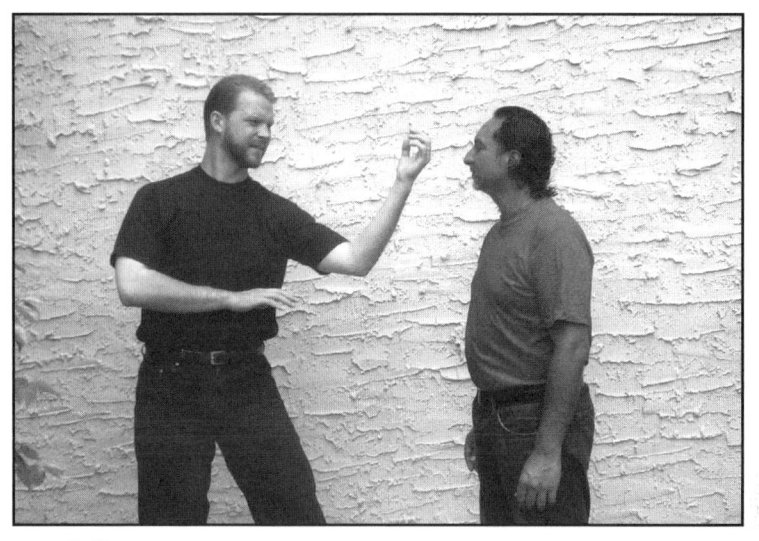

2. Raise your arm upward, extending the elbow forward.

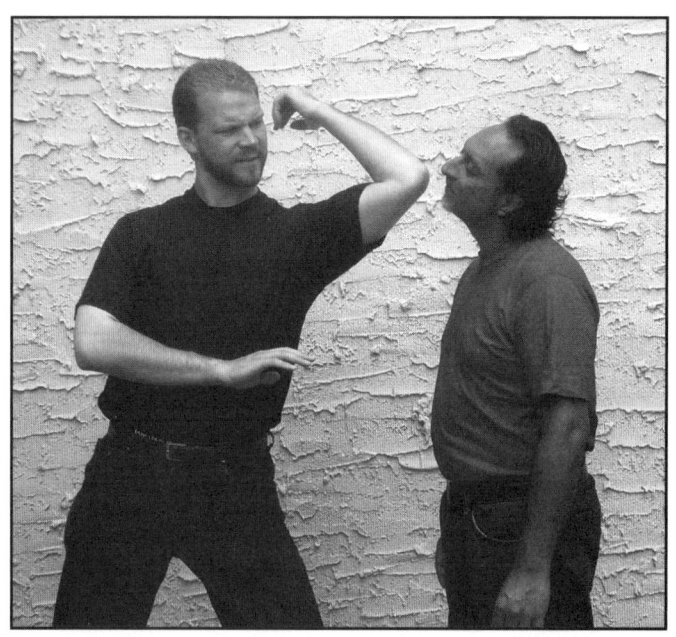

3. Complete the attack by pulling your wrist back and swinging the tip of the elbow to the attacker's face.

HAND & ARM ATTACKS

The very first thing that you must consider when you find yourself in a confrontation is, of course, the maintenance of your personal safety. I have seen far too many foolish people crack their hands punching someone in the skull because they did not follow simple guidelines for effective hand techniques. Remember the one rule that clarifies all: Bone doesn't go against bone.

Never use movements that seem uncomfortable to you. You can only change your confidence in techniques by extensively training the desired moves.

CHAPTER 3
UPPER BODY
MANIPULATIONS

Overcoming the aggression of one's opponent can be achieved in a relatively effortless manner. Having faced many adversaries larger than myself, I had no choice but to use my brains instead of brawn. One night while working at the nightclub "The Gate", I found myself coming to the aid of another security guard who was being attacked by several assailants. Unable to out-muscle them, I used quick body manipulations to nullify their numerical advantage over me. The techniques listed below are among the moves that allowed me to overcome and subdue their aggressions until I received backup.

The object of this chapter is to instruct the reader on how to quickly and easily absorb, manipulate, and redistribute an adversary's energy against them. Whether offensive or defensive, the techniques outlined in this section offer concise explanations of how to react to and take advantage of any attacker. The outlined subdivisions below separate each proper reaction based on opportunity and desired result.

With any attack, the most important thing is to avoid injury. However, due to the unknown strength and skill level of a random opponent, you cannot be sure of your ability to easily block an aggression. Knowing that the stronger man may be the one attacking, you must decide upon an effective way to dispense their assault. By accepting and manipulating an attacker's assault in separate parts, we find that we can distribute the force dealt to us in equal and lesser pieces, rather than accepting 100% of the blow in one shot. Rolling Fists and Tunneling are styles of energy management that produce exactly that result. These techniques prove effective regardless of which side one is attacked on.

Important Note: Rolling fists, both 3-point and 4-point, are used prior to and during contact having been made by either of the fighters. Tunneling deals with situations after the fact. Offensive or defensive, any fighter can gain the body positioning they desire depending on which technique they choose to perform. To more easily identify each situation, we will refer to "Mirror Handed" & "Cross handed" variations.

Mirror Hand

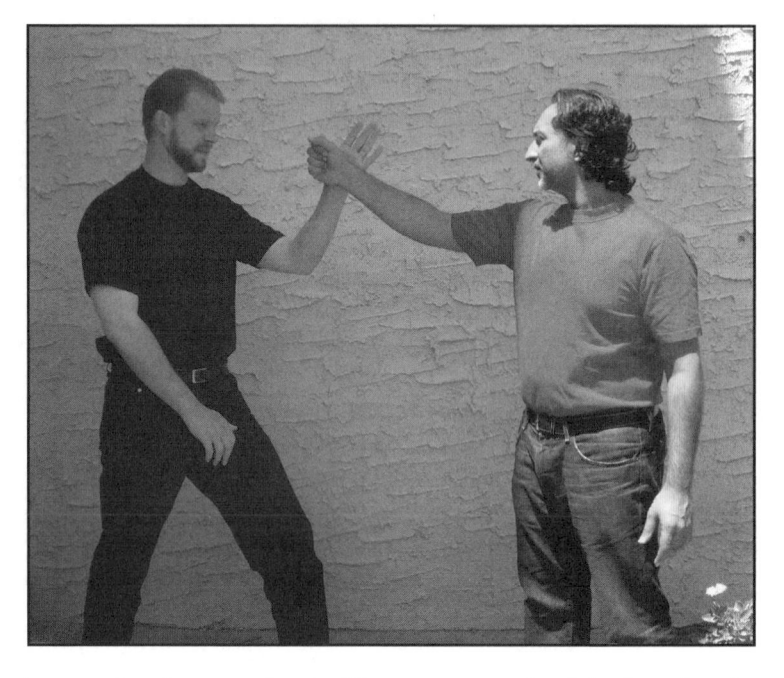

Imagine staring into a mirror. Your opponent's right hand or foot is equally matched by your own left.

UPPER BODY MANIPULATIONS

Cross Hand

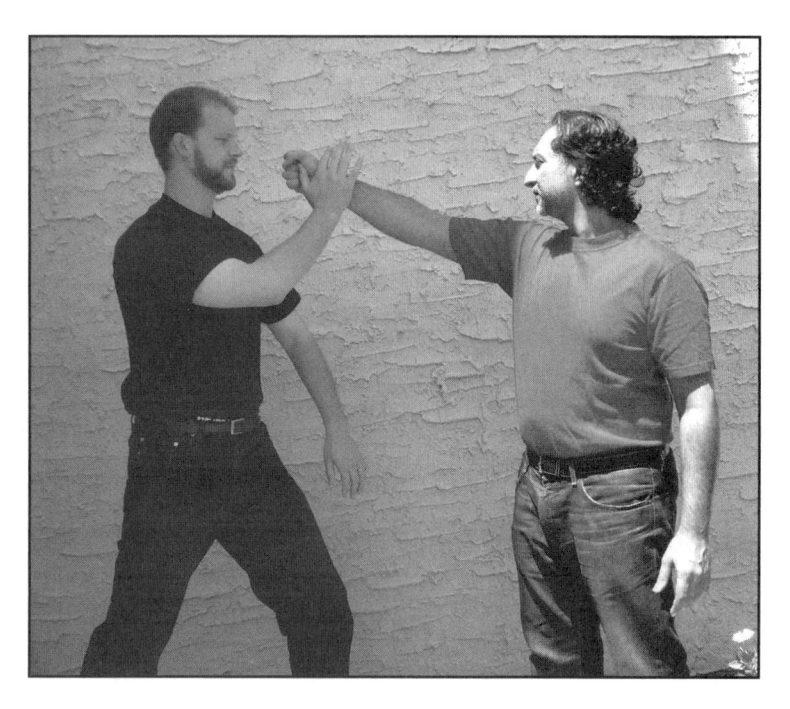

Your opponent's right hand or foot is equally matched across your bodies by your own right hand or foot.

3 Point Rolling Fists

A 3 Point Rolling Fist is executed in order to position one's self free of an opponent's contact after a punch has been thrown. The first and most important movement is, of course, the block. The blocking hand should be positioned with an open palm (See *Chapter 2: Hand and Arm Attacks*), making certain not to block further than 1 inch past your body; once a punch is past you, it can no longer hurt you and there is little point in losing control of the attacking hand once you have begun to manipulate it.

After the first move has successfully been completed, you continue to the second and third part of the technique, "manipulation and redistribution of energy."

Rolling Fists should be performed with open palms for all three movements, but can be interchanged with other hand positioning (See Chapter 2.) Recommended Finishing Strikes will be listed after each heading for suggested final attacks.

Important note: Changing from defense to offense is as simple as moving forward and grabbing (or ripping) with the first move instead of standing still and blocking with it. Simply substitute each initial block in the chosen technique with technique below.

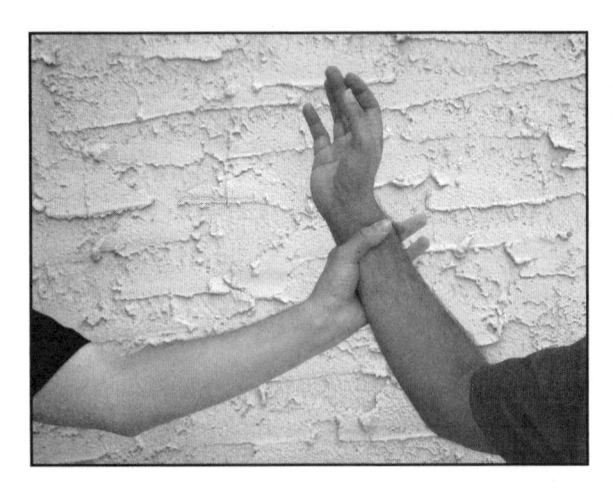

OFFENSIVE SUBSTITUTION FOR MANIPULATION TECHNIQUES

3 Point Outside Rolling Fists

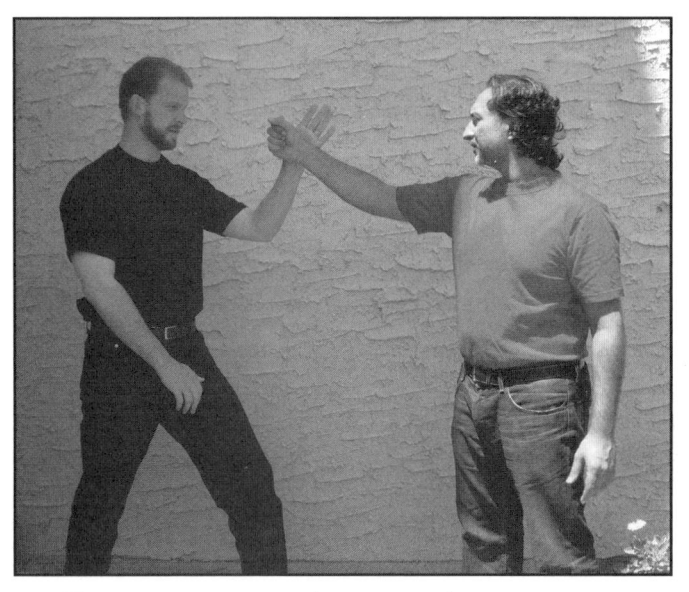

1. Press your open palm (mirror hand) against the outside of the attacker's wrist.

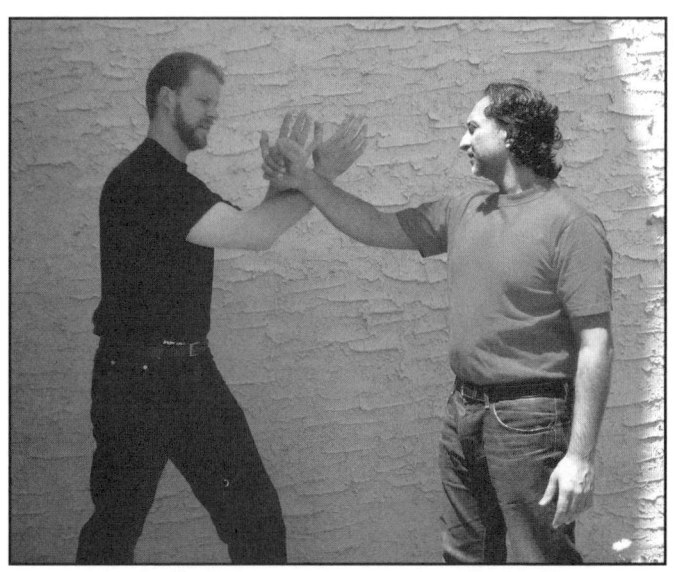

2. Lift your cross hand underneath both of the arms, making firm contact with the opponent's forearm.

UPPER BODY MANIPULATIONS

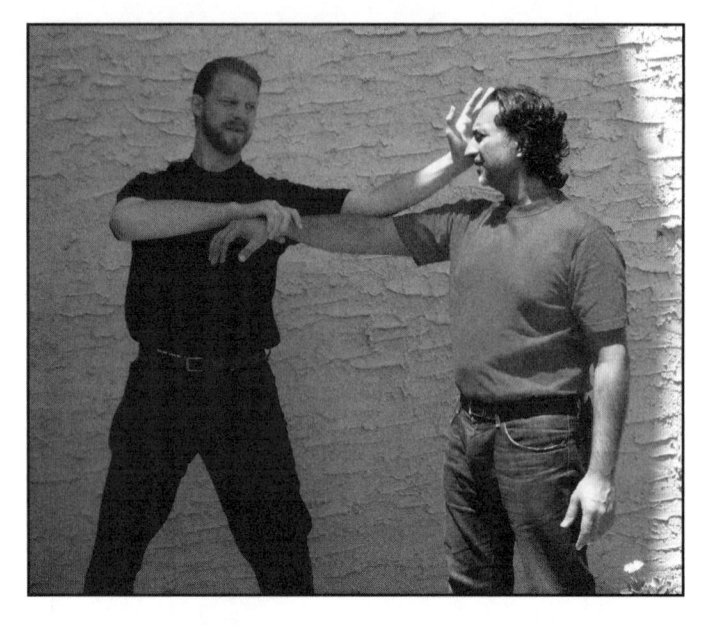

3. Sliding back to grab the opponent's wrist with your cross hand, palm strike the opponent with your free hand.

Recommended Finishing Strikes: Half Fist, Star Fist/Eagles Beak, Palm Strike, Whip Hands, Wrist Strike

3 Point Inside Rolling Fists

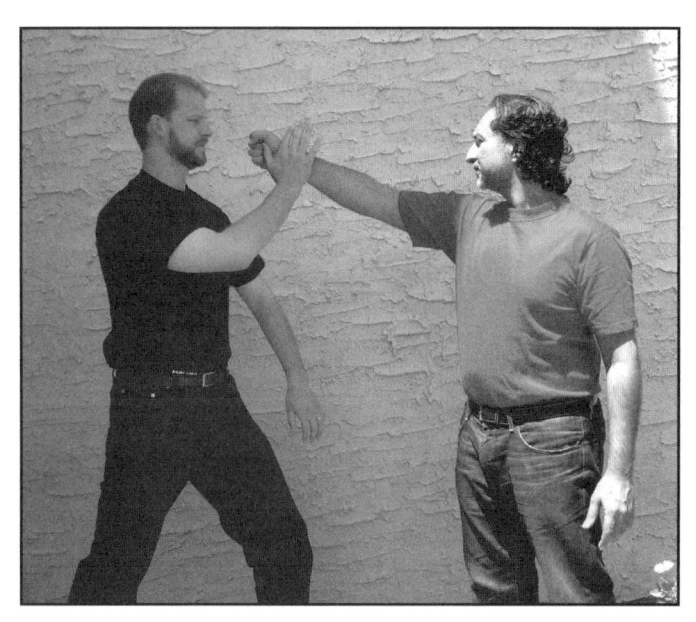

1. Press your open palm (cross hand) against the inside of the attacker's wrist.

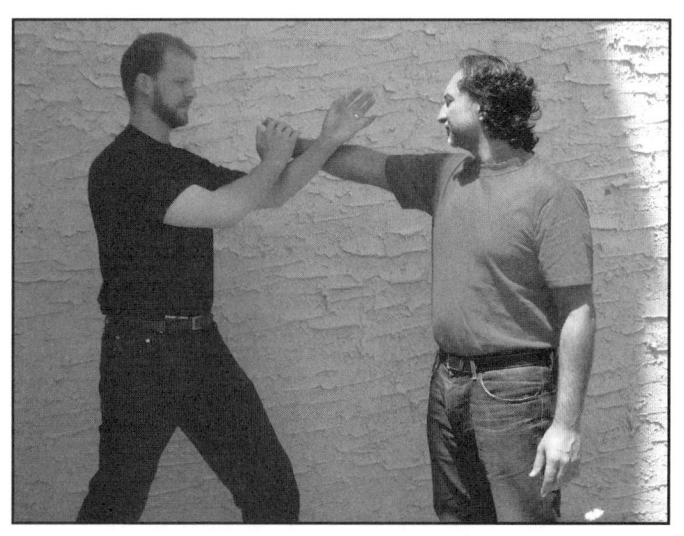

2. Lift your mirror hand underneath both arms, trading control of the opponent's forearm.

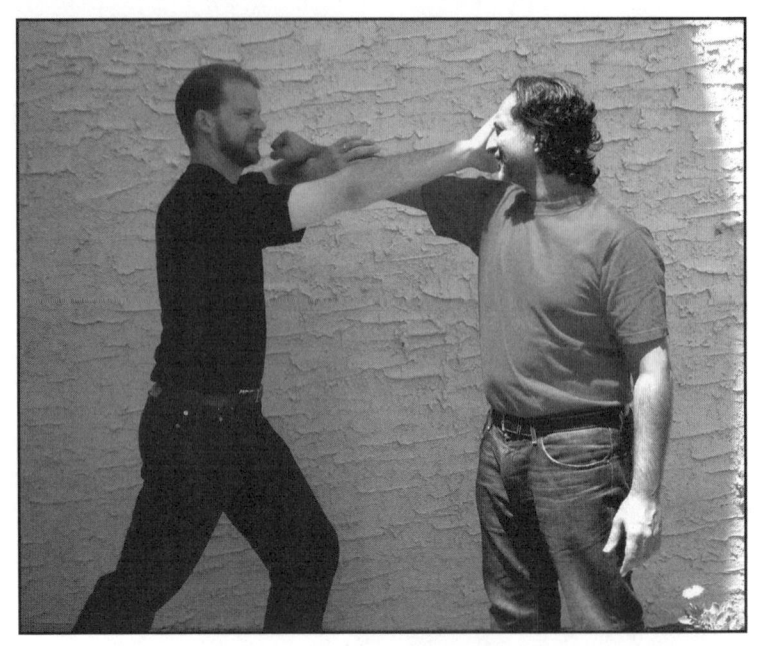

3. PALM STRIKE THE OPPONENT WITH YOUR FREE HAND.

Recommended Finishing Strikes: Back Fist, Finger Gouge, Thumb Spike, Palm Strike, Chop

UPPER BODY MANIPULATIONS

3 Point Upward Rolling Fists

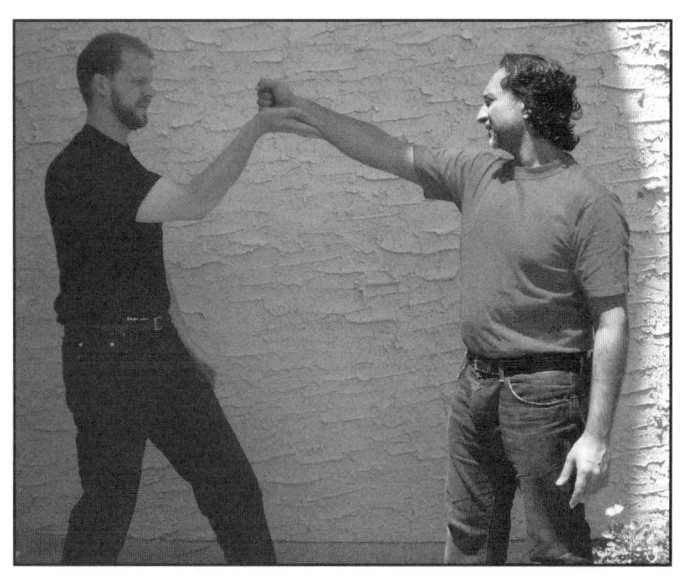

1. Lift the opponent's wrist with the palm of your cross hand.

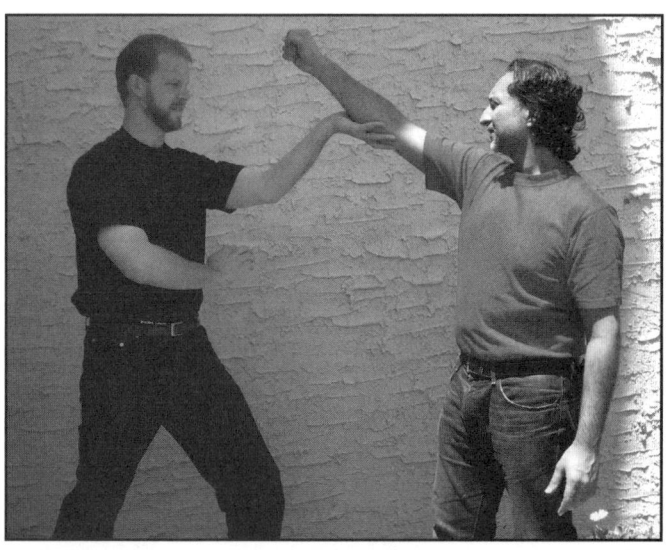

2. Continue forward, lifting just above the opponent's elbow with your mirror hand.

UPPER BODY MANIPULATIONS

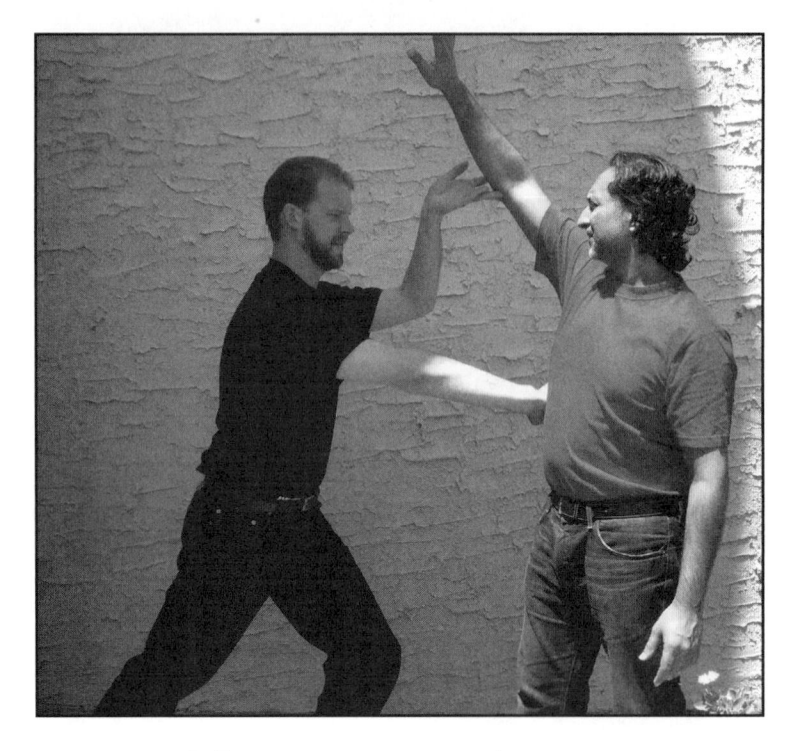

3. Palm strike the opponent's ribcage.

Recommended Finishing Strikes: Half Fist, Back Fist, Star Fist/Eagles Beak, Palm Strike, Acute Angle Elbow Strike

UPPER BODY MANIPULATIONS

3 Point Downward Rolling Fists

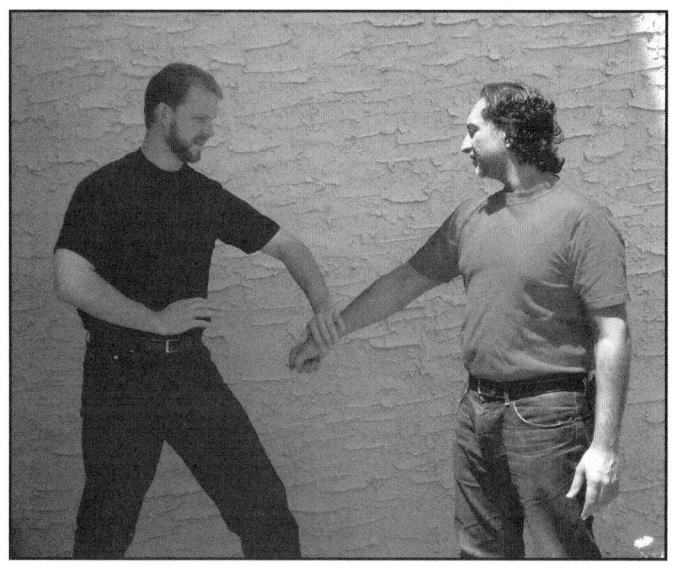

1. PRESS THE OPPONENT'S WRIST AND PULL DOWNWARD WITH YOUR MIRROR HAND.

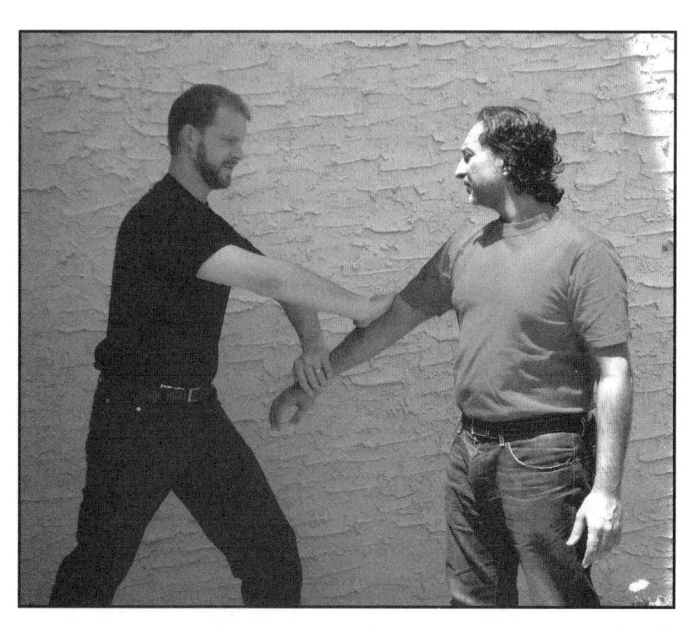

2. CLIMB YOUR CROSS HAND UP THE ATTACKING ARM AND OVER OPPONENT'S ELBOW.

UPPER BODY MANIPULATIONS

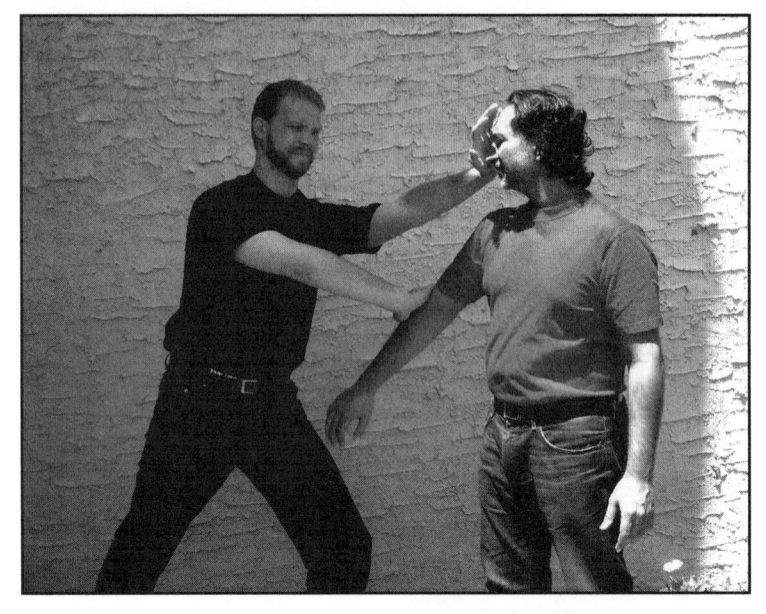

3. Palm strike the opponent with your free hand.

Recommended Finishing Strikes: Whole fist, Finger Gouge, Palm Strike, Claw, Obtuse, Angle Elbow Strike

3 Point Destruction Rolling Fists

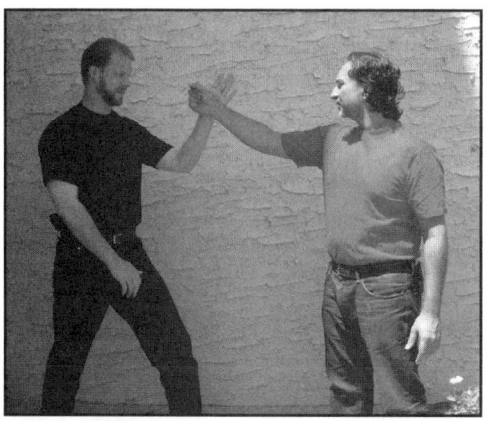

1. PRESS YOUR OPEN PALM (MIRROR HAND) AGAINST THE OUTSIDE OF ATTACKER'S WRIST.

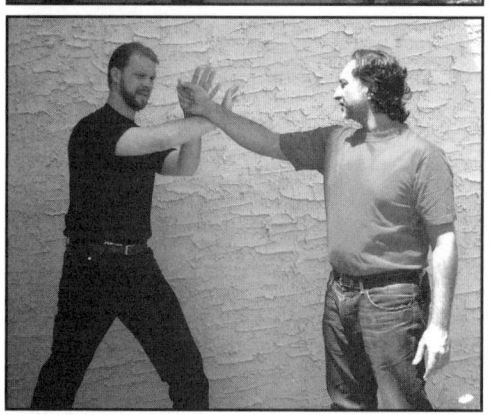

2. LIFT YOUR CROSS HAND UNDERNEATH BOTH ARMS, GRABBING THE OUTSIDE OF OPPONENT'S WRIST.

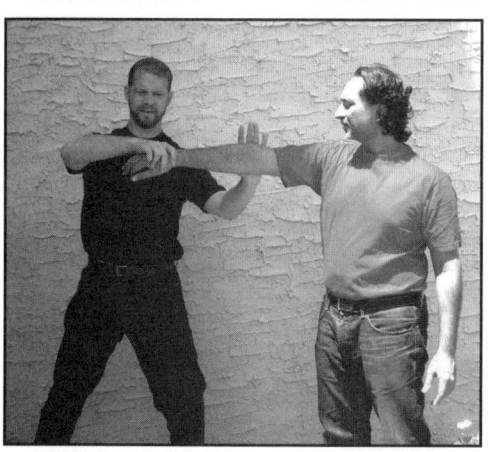

3. MAINTAINING THE GRAB, DESTROY THE OPPONENT'S ELBOW BY PRESSING FIRMLY AGAINST IT WITH YOUR MIRROR HAND.

4 Point Rolling Fists

4 Point Rolling Fists are used when you wish to stay both close and in front of (facing) their opponent while still maintaining contact with the attacker. Similar to 3 Point Rolling Fists, 4 Point Rolling Fists insert a pinning hand as the third movement before attacking.

The same considerations remain relevant for the differential between offense and defense, but the choice of this movement offers the opportunity to choke or tie your opponent while he is still standing. A second's time is all it takes to secure an advantage and 4-point Rolling Fists offer just that.

4 Point Outside Rolling Fists

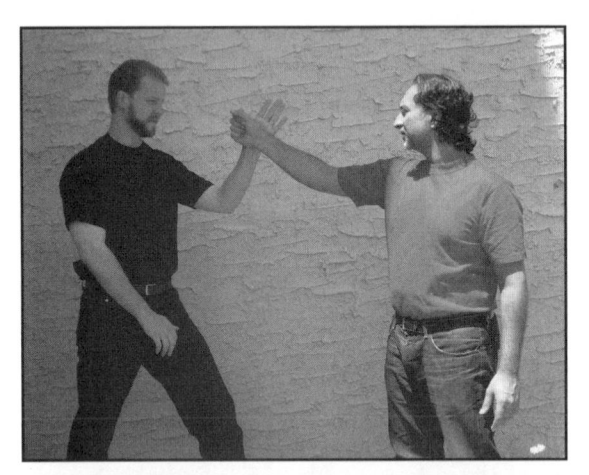

1. PRESS THE OUTSIDE OF THE OPPONENT'S ATTACKING WRIST WITH YOU MIRROR HAND.

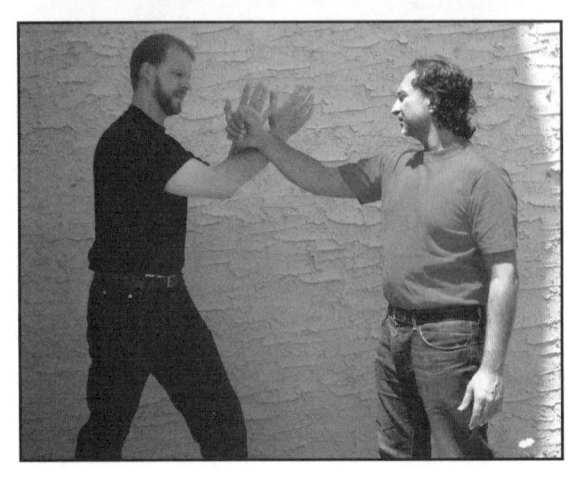

2. LIFT YOUR CROSS HAND UNDERNEATH BOTH ARMS, MAINTAINING FIRM CONTACT WITH THE OPPONENT'S FOREARM.

UPPER BODY MANIPULATIONS

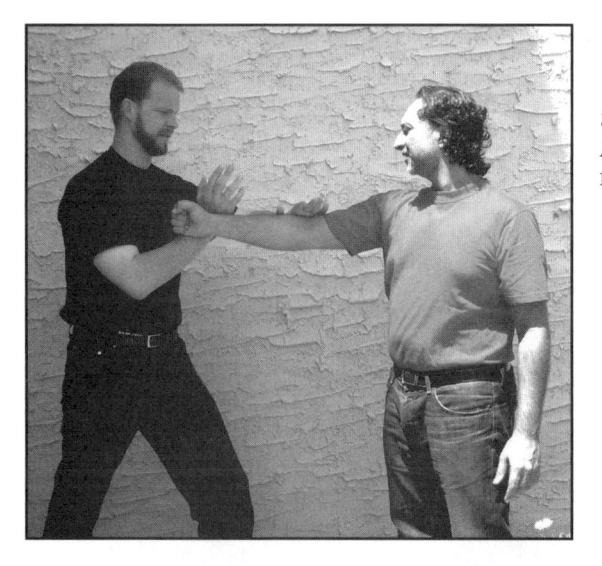

3. CONTROL THE OPPONENT'S ATTACKING ARM WITH YOUR MIRROR HAND.

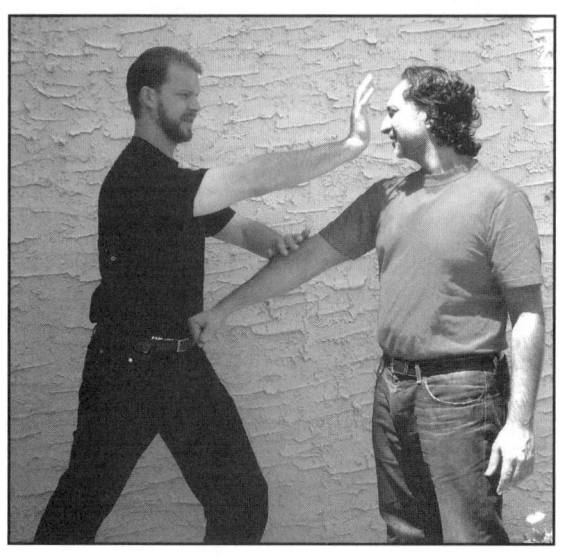

4. STRIKE THE OPPONENT WITH YOUR FREE HAND.

Recommended Finishing Strikes: Half Fist, Finger Gouge, Palm Strike, Knife Hand, Forearm Attack

4 Point Inside Rolling Fists

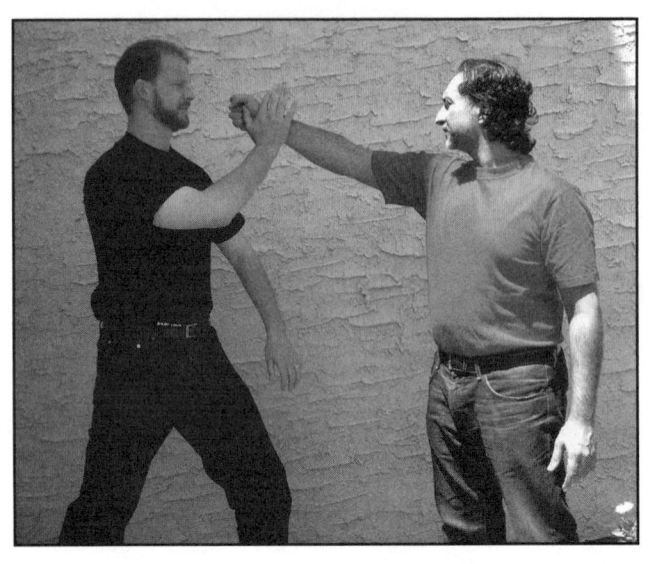

1. Press your open palm (cross hand) against the inside of attacker's wrist.

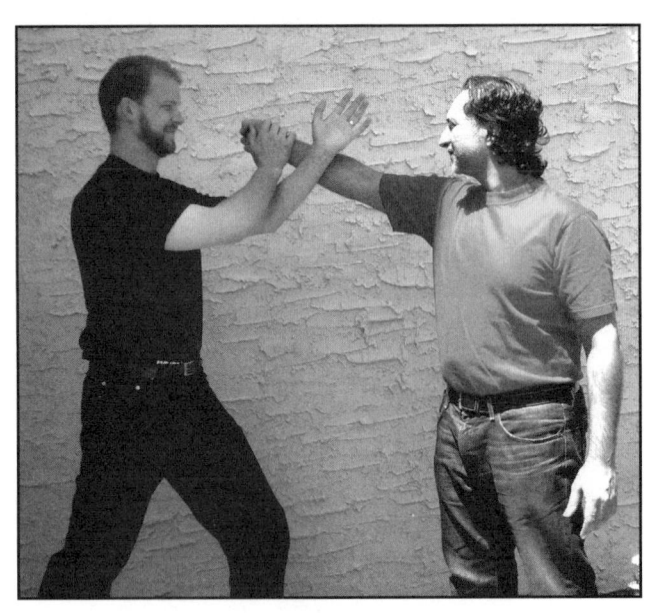

2. Lift your mirror hand underneath both arms, maintaining firm contact with the inside of opponent's forearm.

UPPER BODY MANIPULATIONS

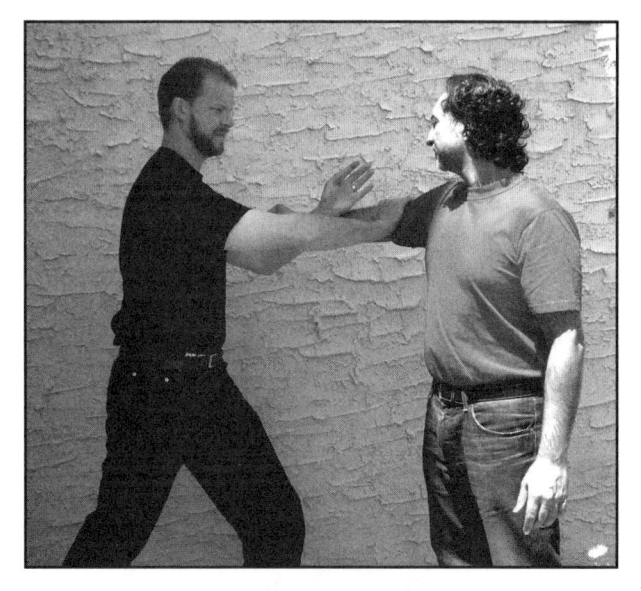

3. CONTROL THE OPPONENT'S ATTACKING ARM WITH YOUR CROSS HAND.

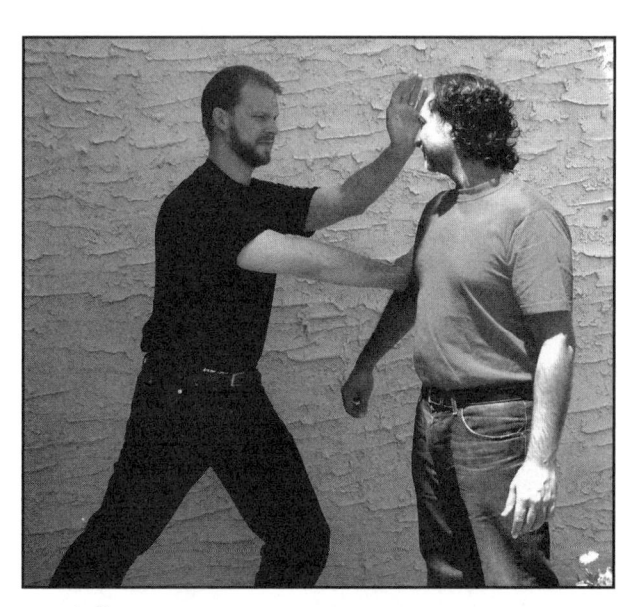

4. STRIKE THE OPPONENT WITH YOUR FREE HAND.

Recommended Finishing Strikes: Star Fist/Eagles Beak, Finger Gouge, Thumb Spike, Palm Strike, Claw, Whip Hands, Chop

4 Point Bridge (Upward) Rolling Fists

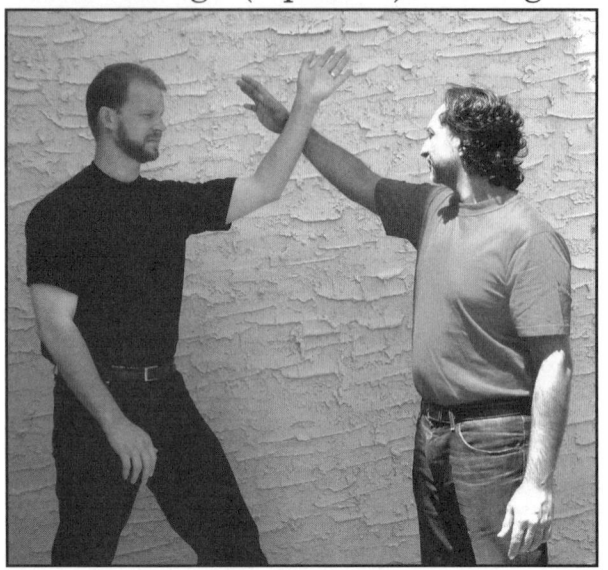

1. Block the attacker's strike with the outside of your mirror hand forearm.

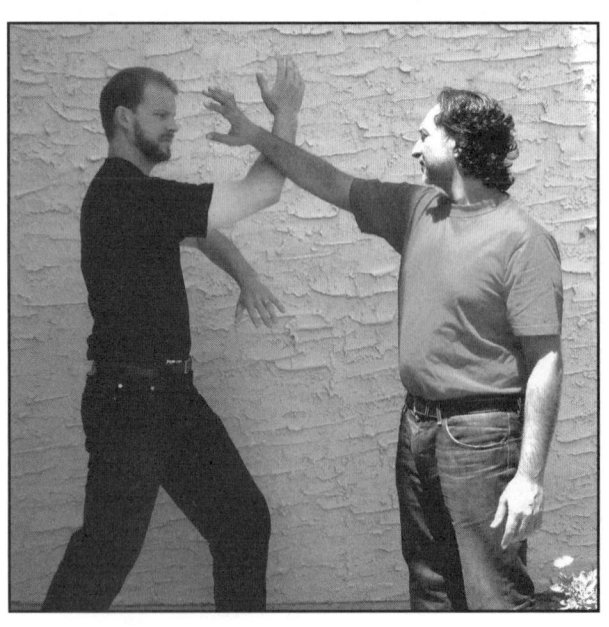

2. Lift your cross hand underneath both arms, trading contact of the opponent's attack from one arm to the other.

UPPER BODY MANIPULATIONS

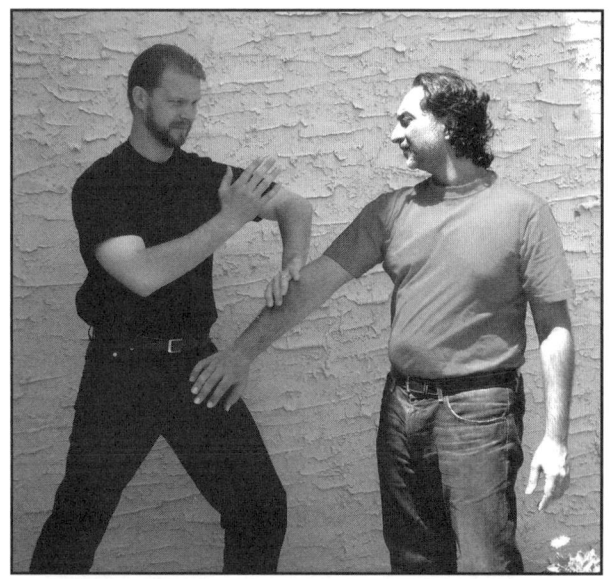

3. CONTROL THE OPPONENT'S ATTACKING ARM DOWNWARD WITH YOUR MIRROR HAND.

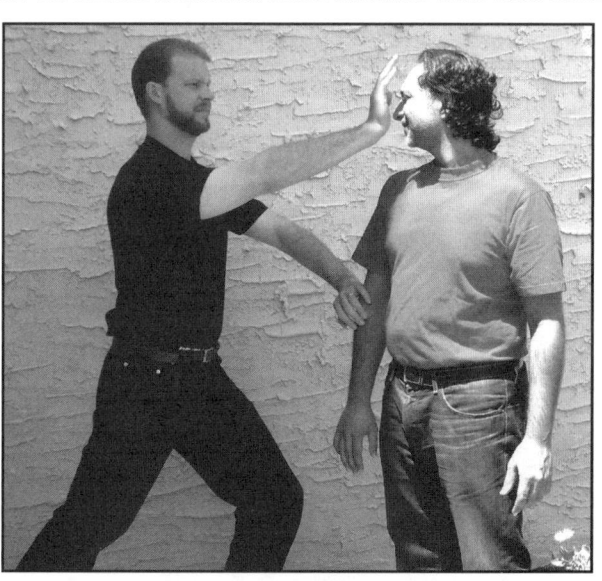

4. STRIKE THE OPPONENT WITH YOUR FREE HAND.

Recommended Finishing Strikes: Finger Gouge, Palm Strike, Knife Hand, Wrist Attack, Forearm Attack, Obtuse Angle Elbow Strike

4 Point Downward Rolling Fists

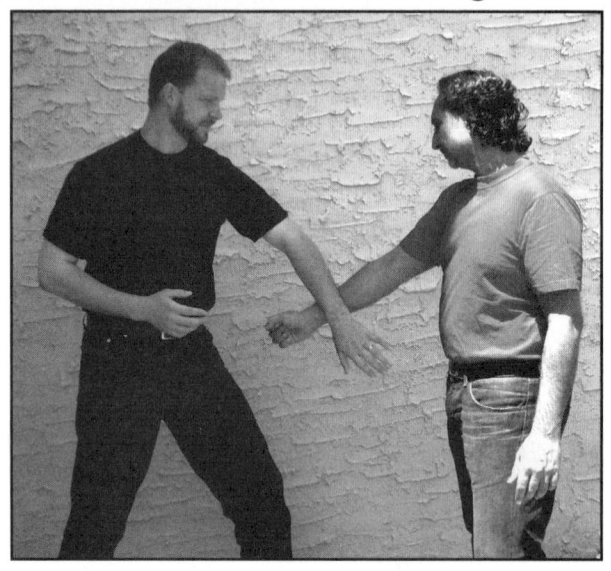

1. BLOCK THE OPPONENT'S FOREARM DOWNWARD WITH THE INSIDE OF YOUR MIRROR HAND FOREARM.

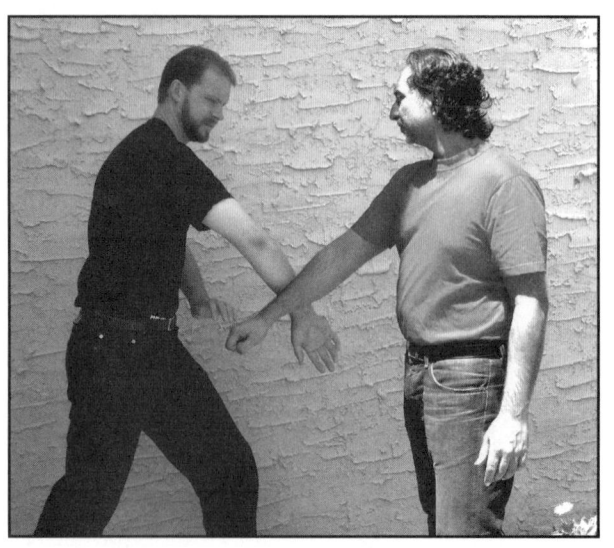

2. PRESS YOUR CROSS HAND OVER BOTH ARMS, MAINTAINING FIRM CONTACT WITH THE OPPONENT'S ATTACKING FOREARM.

UPPER BODY MANIPULATIONS

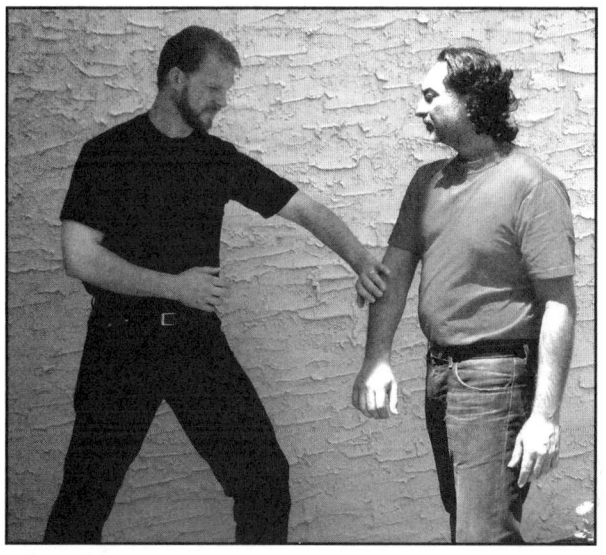

3. PRESS THE OPPONENT'S ATTACKING ARM AGAINST HIS BODY WITH YOUR MIRROR HAND.

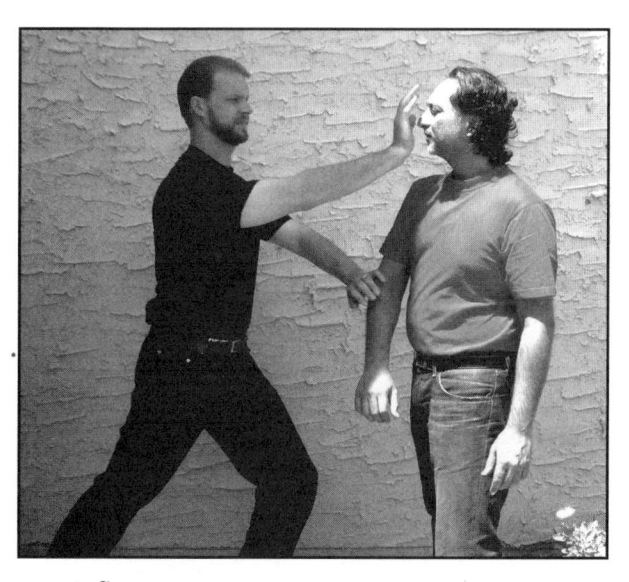

4. STRIKE THE OPPONENT WITH YOUR FREE HAND.

Recommended Finishing Strikes: Finger Gouge, Palm Strike, Knife Hand, Wrist Attack, Forearm Attack, Obtuse Angle Elbow Strike

UPPER BODY MANIPULATIONS

4 Point Destruction Rolling Fists

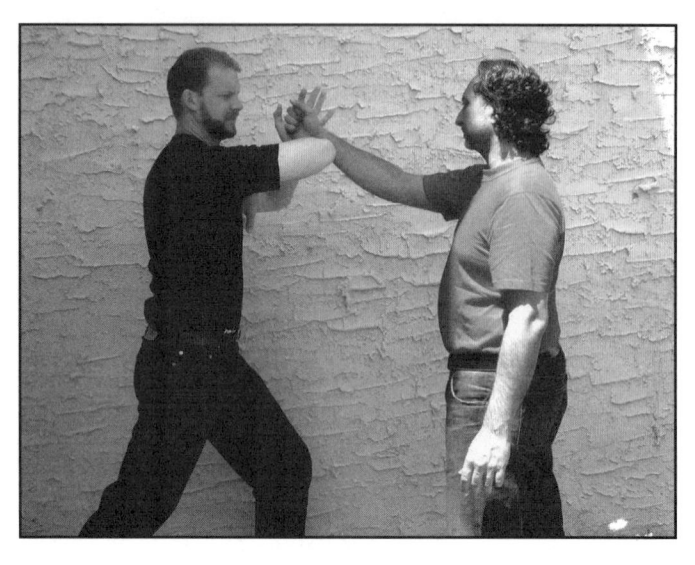

1. PRESS YOUR OPEN PALM (MIRROR HAND) AGAINST THE OUTSIDE OF ATTACKER'S WRIST AND SLAM A CROSS HANDED ELBOW AGAINST THE INSIDE OF OPPONENT'S WRIST.

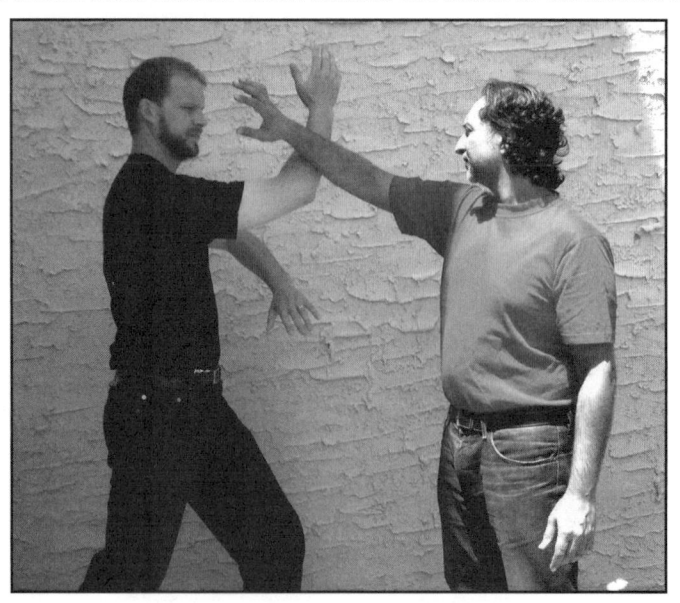

2. CONTINUE BY LIFTING YOUR CROSS HAND UNDERNEATH BOTH ARMS, CONTINUING FIRM CONTACT WITH THE OPPONENT'S FOREARM.

UPPER BODY MANIPULATIONS

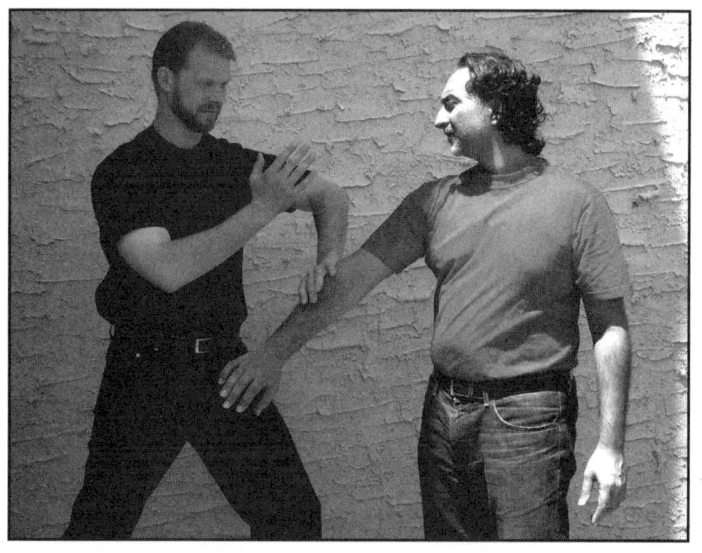

3. Control the opponent's attacking arm downward with your mirror hand.

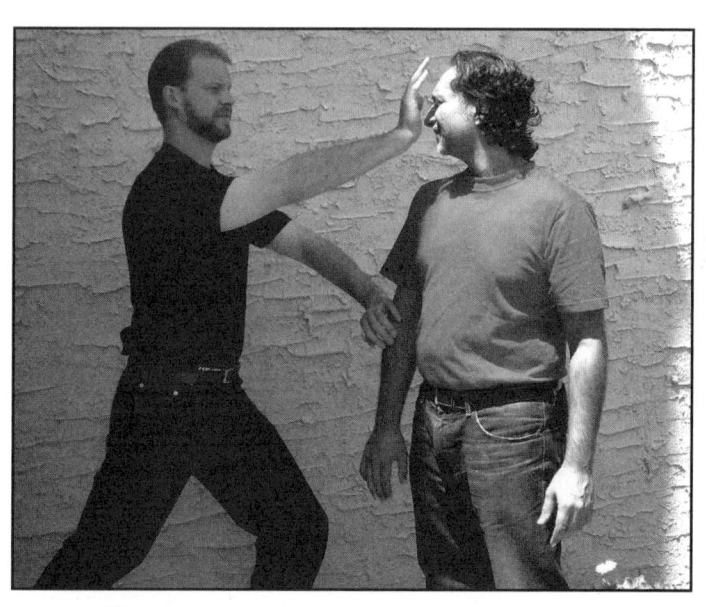

4. Strike the opponent with your free hand.

Recommended Finishing Strikes: Finger Gouge, Palm Strike, Knife Hand, Wrist Attack, Forearm Attack, Obtuse Angle Elbow Strike

Tunneling

Within the myriad of situations that arise after contact with the opposition has been made, we find ourselves with two equally effective choices; maintaining or dissolving contact. Tunneling utilizes touch sensitivity and steady contact with the opponent to detect their weaknesses and vulnerabilities as well as acting upon these once they are revealed. Whether contact has been made with one or both hands, tunneling enables one to garner advantage while preserving safety. Decisive movement makes it easy to choke or tie up one's opponent, leaving striking opportunities almost limitless.

In this section we will focus on three easy to understand and perform styles of tunneling. During these manipulations, whether mirror or cross handed, it is best to remember to stay directly in front of your opponent, keeping both sets of shoulders square at all times. Training techniques should include practicing with a partner. Make certain to keep constant contact with your partner's wrists. To clarify contact, the push position is illustrated below. (Full body situations will be covered in *Chapter 6: Locks, Grappling,* and *Freeing & Chapter 7: Stepping, Trapping, & Sweeping.*)

Push Position

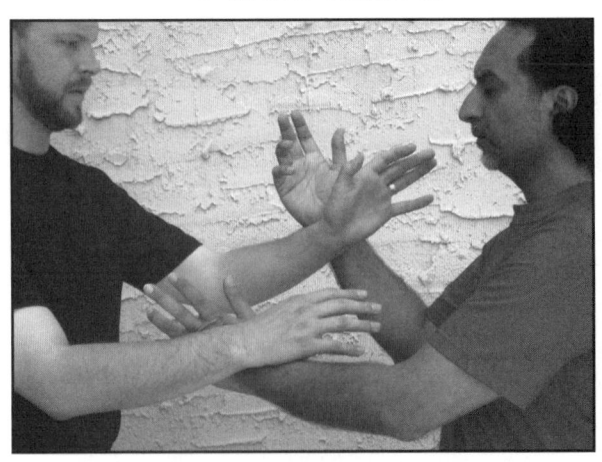

Facing your opponent, force your hands forward into his guard and place them wrist to wrist, one on the inside of your opponent's hand and the other outside. This position assures effective training on both fronts regardless of which party has control of the inside or outside.

UPPER BODY MANIPULATIONS

Double Hand Tunneling

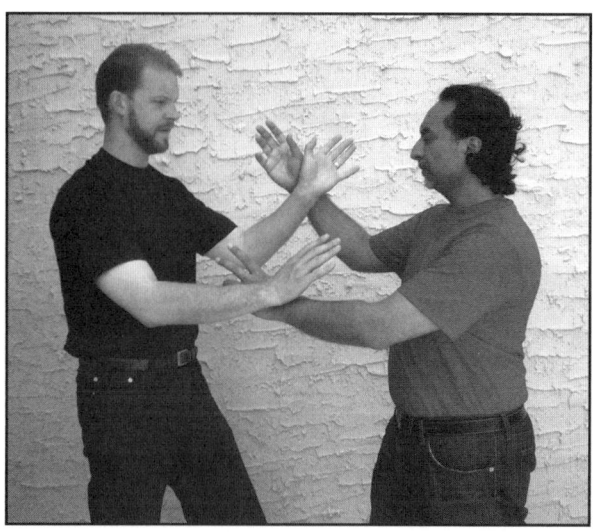

1. Jump into the opponent's hands with a standard "push position"

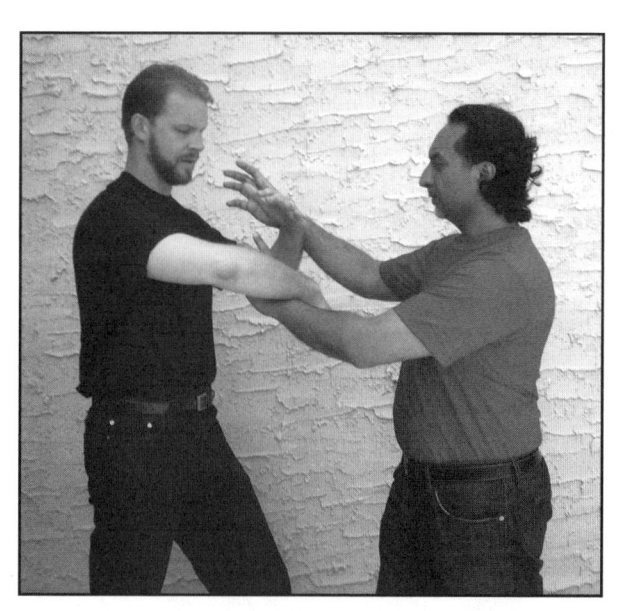

2. Press your right wrist over and atop your opponent's left, pushing it down slightly.

UPPER BODY MANIPULATIONS

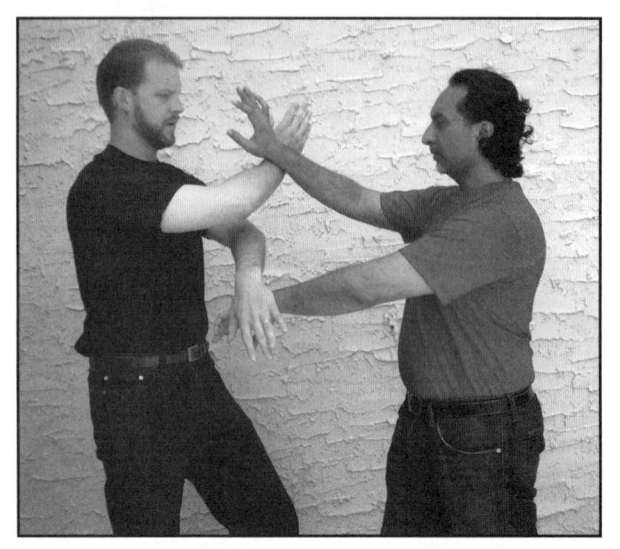

3. Quickly switch the control of your opponent's hands from mirror to cross hands. To do this cup your left hand downward over your opponent's left wrist. **Make sure that these hands stay closest to your own body.** Next, raise your right hand from underneath to grab the outside of your opponent's right wrist.

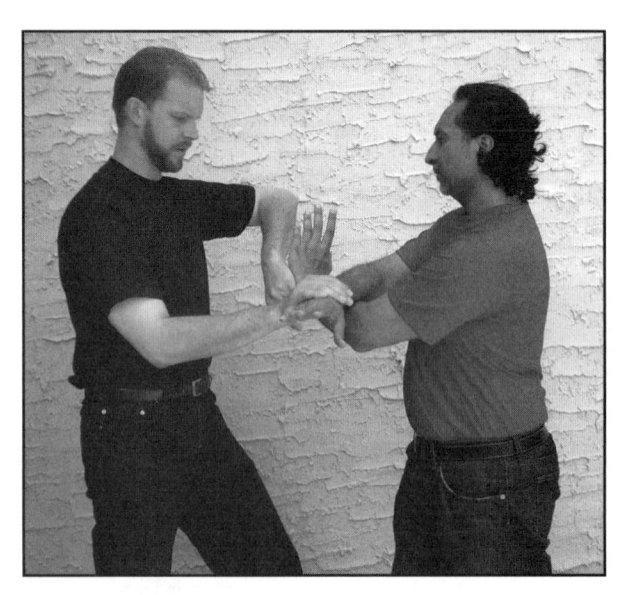

4. After grabbing your attacker's right wrist, pull it down and across his body, pinning his arms together.

UPPER BODY MANIPULATIONS

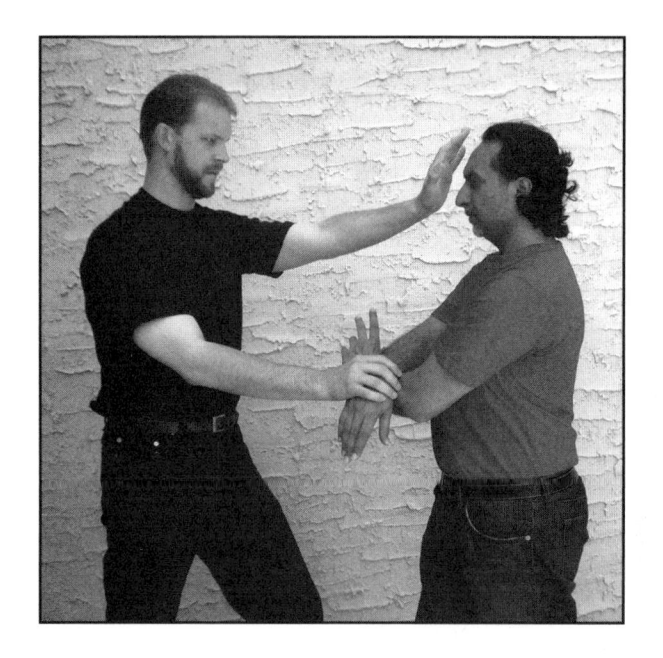

5. STRIKE WITH LEFT HAND.

Recommended Finishing Strikes: Half Fist, Finger Gouge, Palm Strike, Wrist Attack, Forearm Attack, Obtuse Angle Elbow Strike

UPPER BODY MANIPULATIONS

The next two techniques are considered offensive and used only in cross handed situations when the push position cannot be achieved.

Single Hand Entry

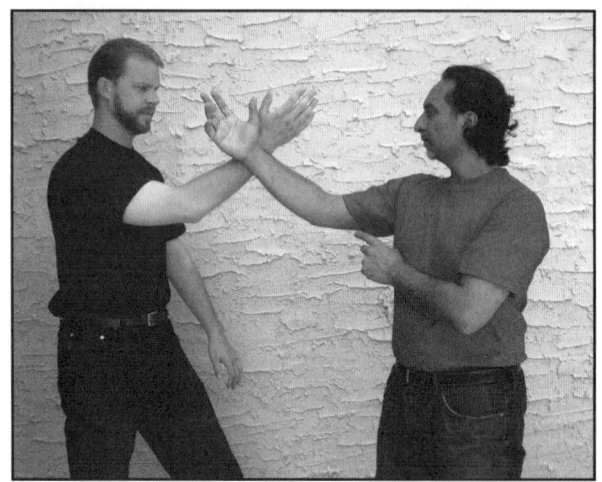

1. RAISE YOUR CROSS HAND, BLOCKING OR ENTERING WITH OUTSIDE WRIST TO WRIST CONTACT WITH THE OPPONENT.

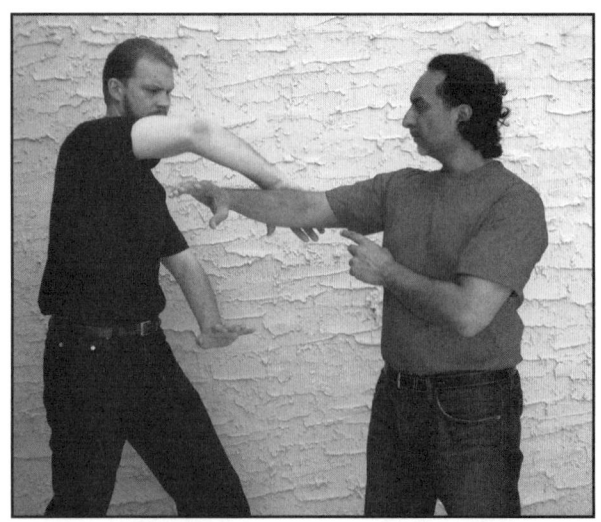

2. SWINGING YOUR ELBOW HIGH, CARRY YOUR HAND DOWN AND CUP THE OPPONENT'S ELBOW, CONTROLLING IT AWAY FROM YOU.

UPPER BODY MANIPULATIONS

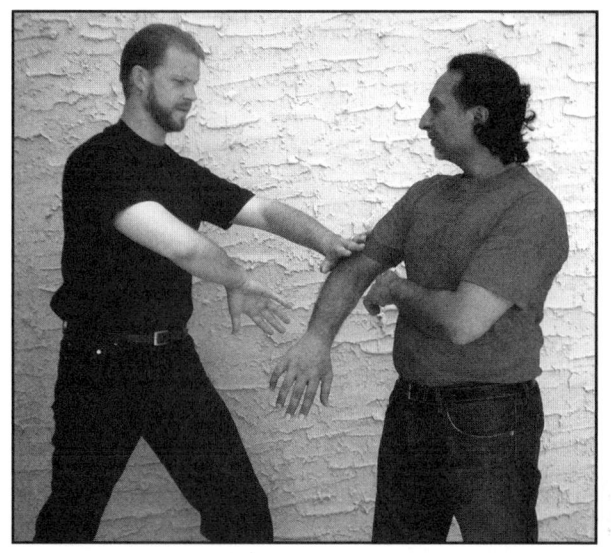

3. Press your mirror hand over the opponent's elbow.

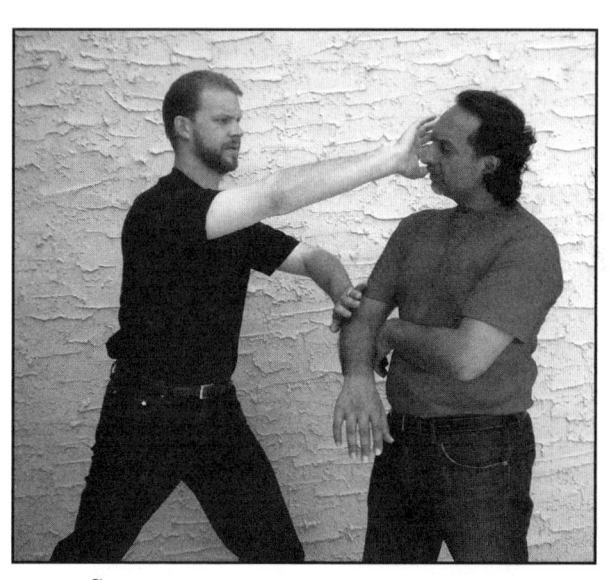

4. Strike the opponent with your free hand.

Recommended Finishing Strikes: Back Fist, Palm Strike, Obtuse Angle Elbow Strike, Acute Angle Elbow Strike

UPPER BODY MANIPULATIONS

Forward Pullback

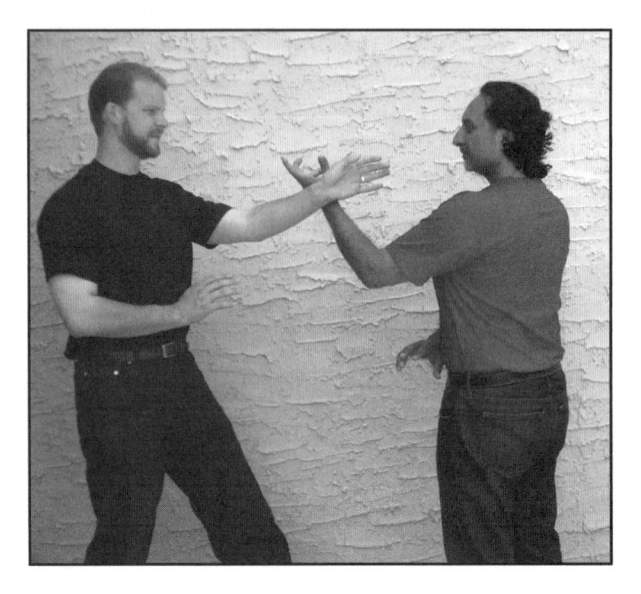

1. Make cross-handed contact at the outside of your wrist and your opponent's wrists, making sure to tip your hand back.

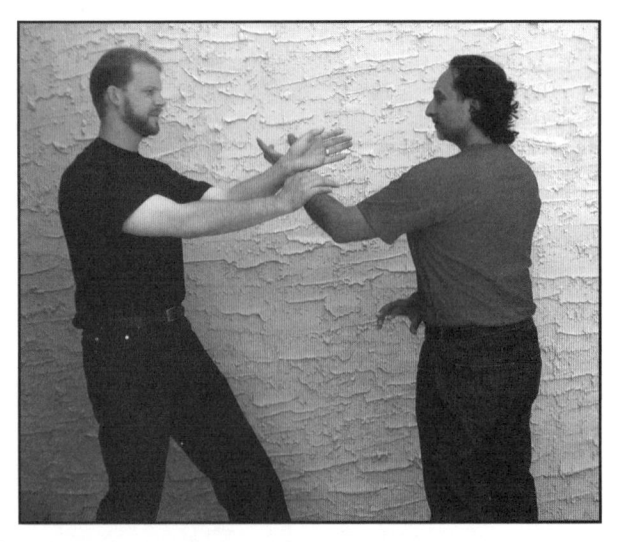

2. Quickly grab the opponent's forearm with your mirror hand.

UPPER BODY MANIPULATIONS

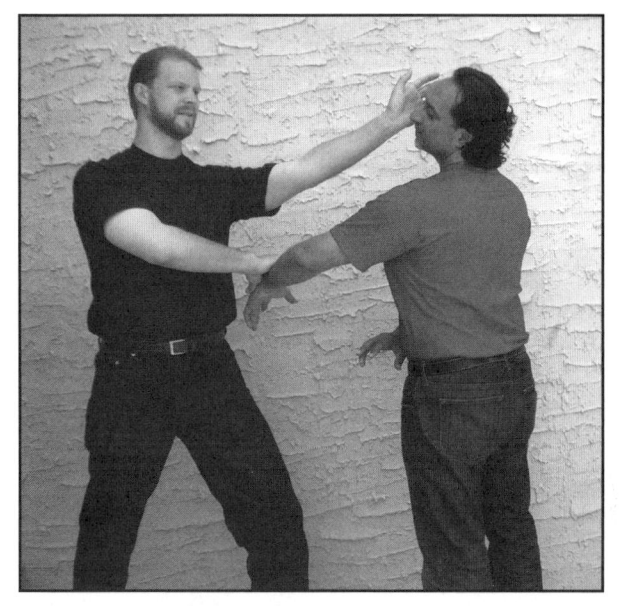

3. Pull the opponent's attacking arm down and strike forward with your cross hand.

Recommended Finishing Strikes: Half Fist, Back Fist, Palm Strike

UPPER BODY MANIPULATIONS

Spreading Waves / Double Handed Push

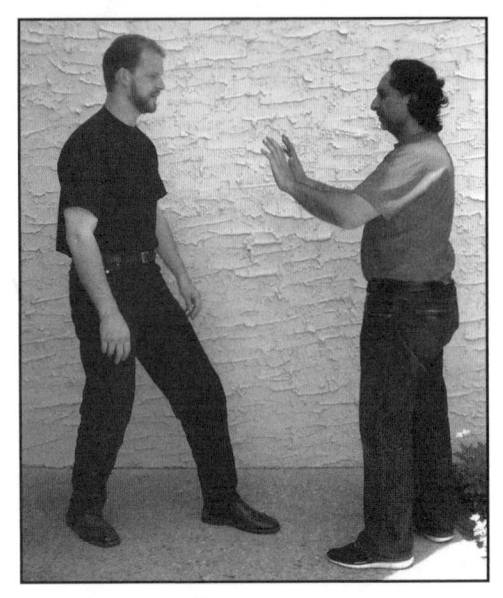

1. THE ATTACKER MOVES TO PUSH AGAINST YOU.

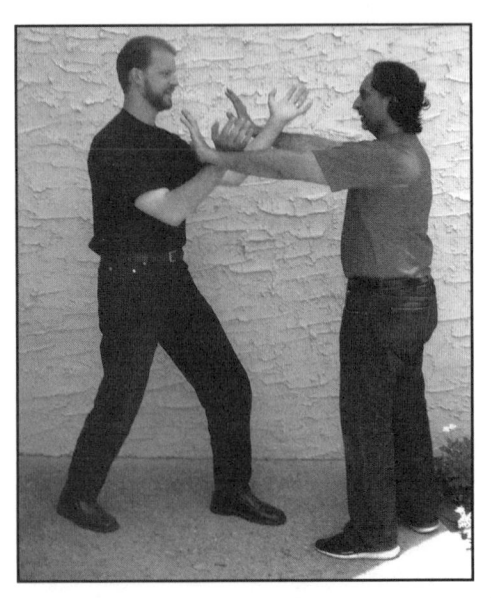

2. RAISE YOUR HANDS UPWARD BETWEEN THE OPPONENT'S ARMS, PUSHING SLIGHTLY WITH YOUR OUTWARD BENT WRISTS.

UPPER BODY MANIPULATIONS

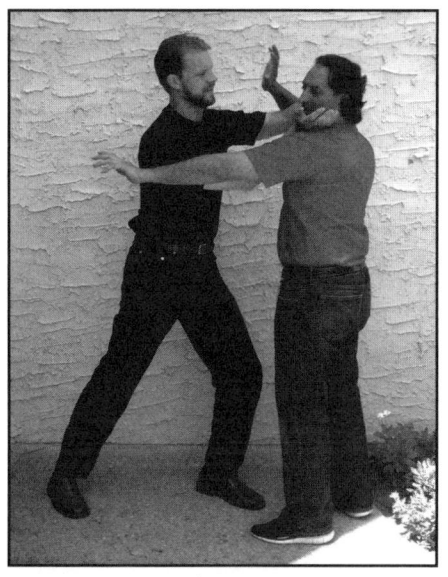

3. After splitting your opponent's hands apart, move quickly inward and place one hand firmly over your attacker's chin and the the other tightly grasping the base of his skull.

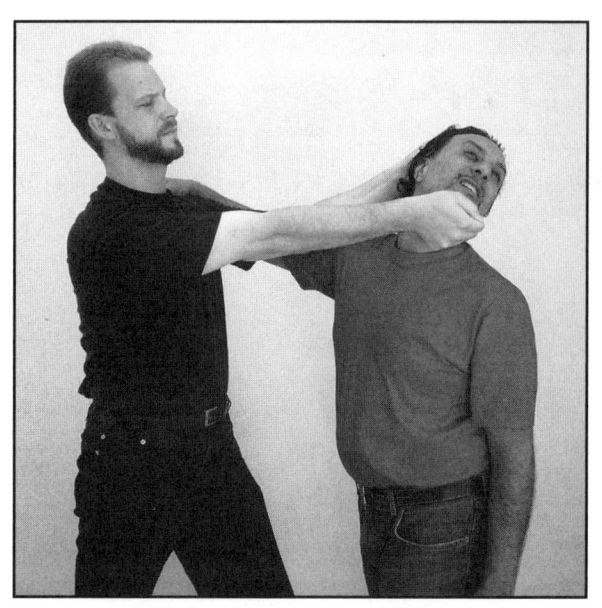

4. Pressing against his chin, twist your opponent's head away from you until a clear advantage is gained.

Once any manipulation technique has been performed, remember that this has been **only one** movement in the fight. As many times as I have witnessed altercations, I watched as the attackers completed one semi-successful move and stood free, foolishly thinking that the fight was over. Take advantage of your opposition's lack of knowledge and experience at every opportunity. Continuous use of the other lessons in this book will allow you to maintain your advantage until the conflict is finished. Remember: Don't stop until victory has been clearly established.

No matter how complicated any technique seems at first, if you practice regularly it will become second nature.

Important Safety Information: If you ever find yourself on the wrong side of a body manipulation, remember that the same rules apply here as they do in other areas of defense. SEPARATE YOURSELF IMMEDIATELY FROM THE DANGER AND START AGAIN!

To achieve the proper release technique when your opponent's upper body manipulation has given him the advantage, simply follow one of the three methods that follow:

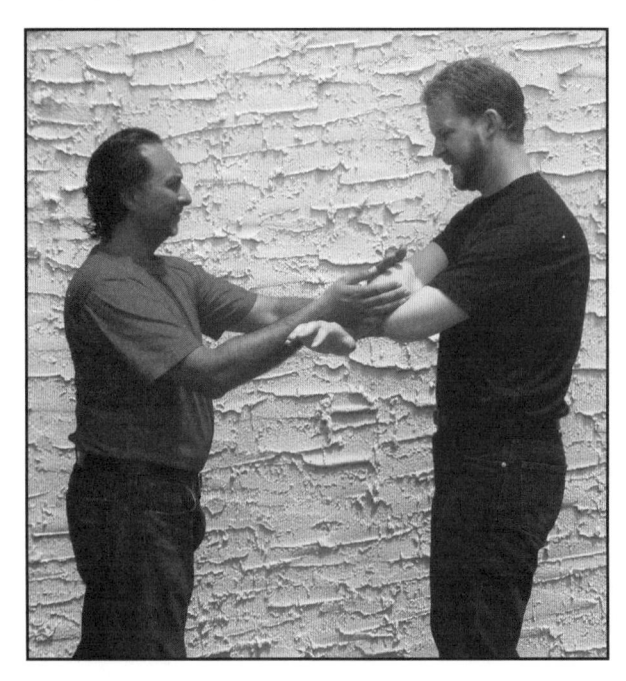

THE OPPONENT HAS TAKEN CONTROL OF MANIPULATION.

Kick Separation

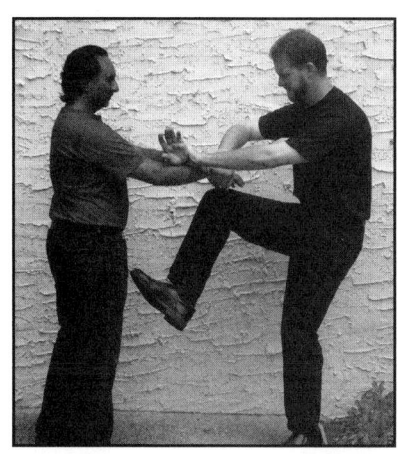

1. LIFT YOUR NEAR LEG UPWARD AT THE KNEE.

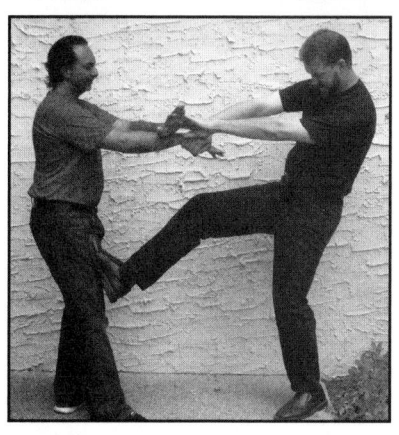

2. PRESS FIRMLY AGAINST THE OPPONENT'S THIGH FOR DISTANCE.

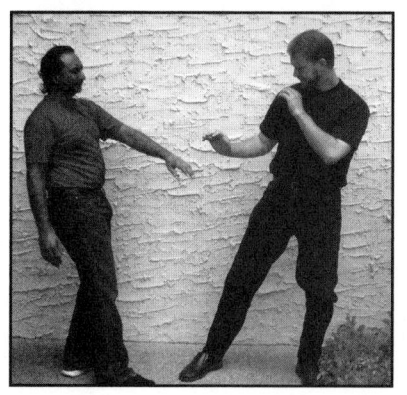

3. SEPARATE, RESET, AND READY FOR A CONTINUED ATTACK.

UPPER BODY MANIPULATIONS

Push Separation

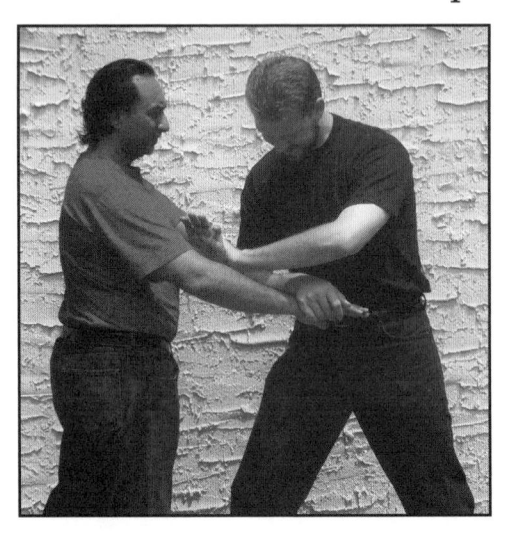

1. Move your shoulders inward, choking the opponent's manipulation.

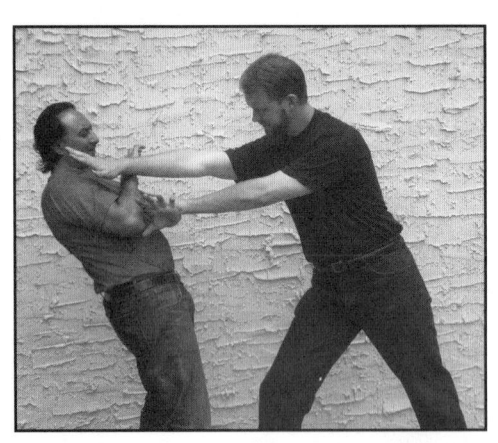

2. Continue applying forward pressure by forcing your hands against the opponent.

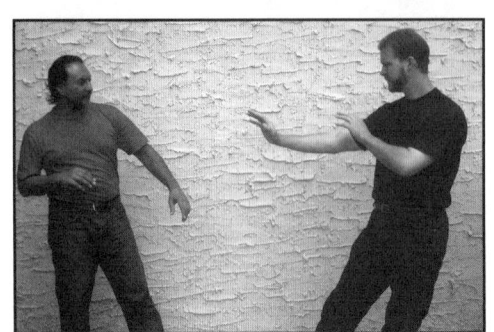

3. Separate, reset, and ready for continued attack.

UPPER BODY MANIPULATIONS

Bump Separation

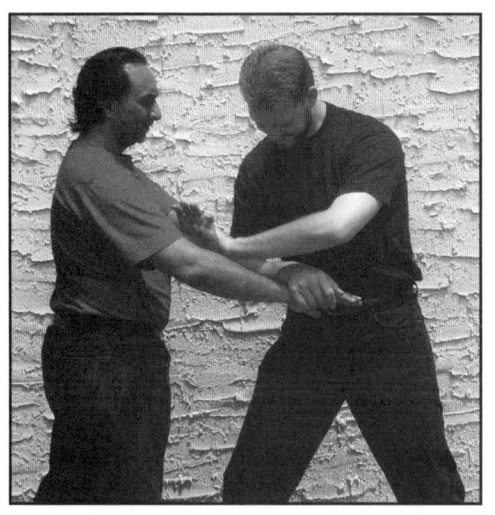

1. Move your shoulders inward, choking opponent's manipulation.

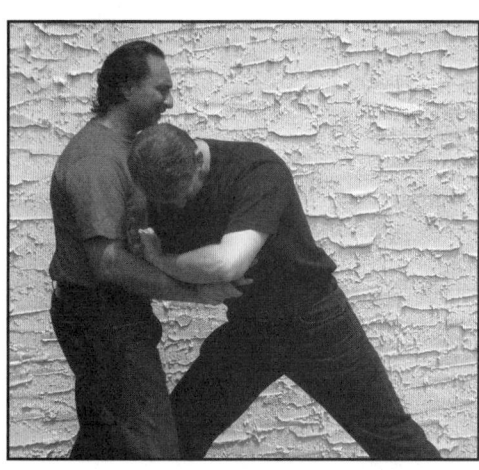

2. Land your shoulder into the opponent, forcing your whole bodyweight against them.

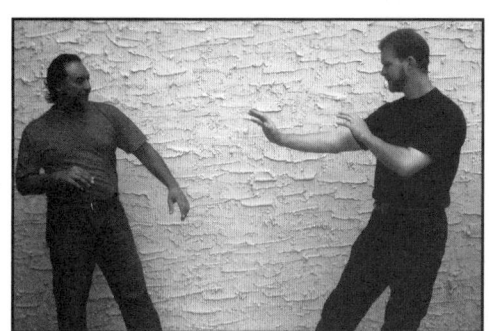

3. Separate, reset, and ready for continued attack.

FOOT AND LEG ATTACKS

CHAPTER 4
FOOT & LEG ATTACKS

One of the most surprising things that I ever witnessed during my time as a bouncer was during an emergency security call. Security staff was forbidden to leave the building in order to handle fights that occurred outside on the sidewalk or parking lot. This rule was however superseded one night when two of the club's bouncers were being attacked by numerous assailants while walking a patron to her car. Having called for help on their radios, every nearby bouncer rushed to give aid. Along with two other members of the security team, I ran swiftly to their location. What happened next was one of the worst brawls I have ever been a part of, but one particular vision stands out in my memory the most.

One of the men who had run outside with me, a man who had a similar martial arts background to my own, chose to throw a high roundhouse kick to an attacker's head. Unfortunately, this imprudent colleague of mine had unwittingly stood himself in a small pool of motor oil and before realizing it, had found himself on his back, in pain, and with a mob of angered club-goers quickly on top of him.

Whether stepping, trapping, or kicking, remember the lesson of this unfortunate bouncer and keep all leg movement below the opponent's waist. Regardless of your level of skill and dexterity, training, or preference for high kicks, the risk is **never** worth it. My colleague learned that lesson the hard way. Low-level kicks are effective and beneficial to the goal of defense. High-level kicks, though extremely powerful, are difficult to land at best. Though offering defense of the upper body by the sheer distance they create, high kicks also risk grave exposure of the groin, knee, and ankle area. Anyone who thinks that these are less vital areas has never taken a knee shot in a fight and found themselves completely immobilized afterwards.

Low-level kicks maintain balance and posture; if for no other reason that should be enough. I have won many a fight by landing a swift kick to the shin or knee. Many types of kicks are effective in close combat. Listed below are several kicking options with full descrip-

Proper Kicking Areas of the Foot

Anyone having ever stubbed their toe even once in their life knows how painful and debilitating this minor injury can be. Consider the abject pain intensified by about ten when you think of a broken foot. There are 26 bones in the human foot. However strong and resilient the feet are, you have to realize that separating the inner bones from one another may be entirely unavoidable if proper kicking techniques are not observed. Kick incorrectly and you may have just won your opponent's victory for them. In order to maintain the safety of your feet during kicking, only certain areas should be used for attack.

Heel Attack

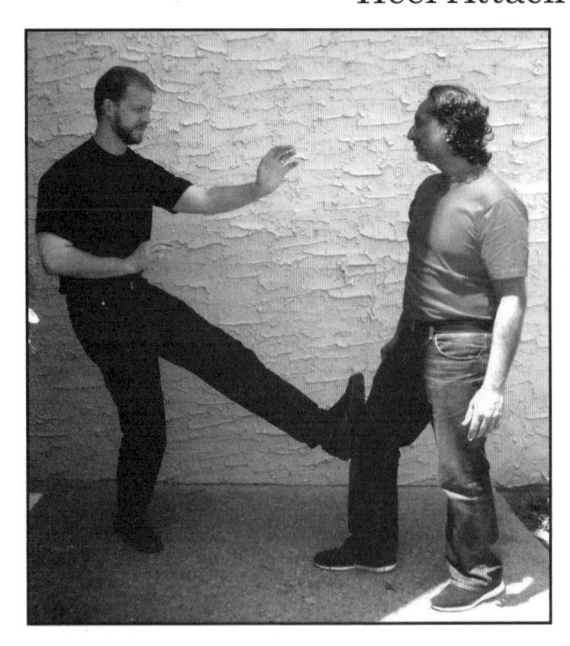

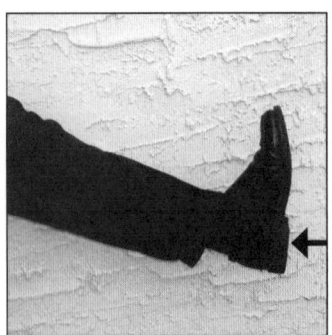

Striking with the heel.

FOOT AND LEG ATTACKS

Ball of Foot Attack

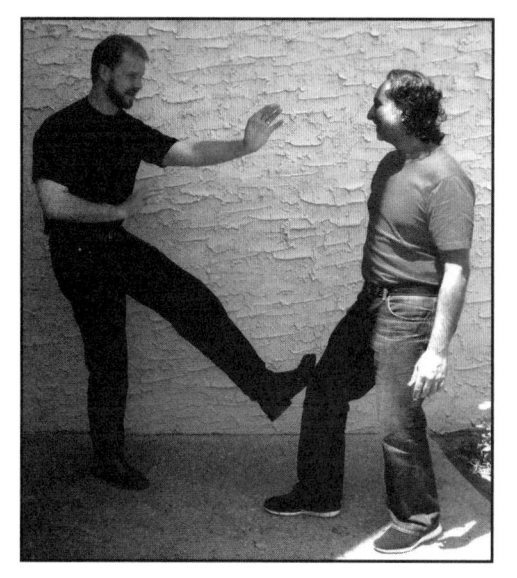

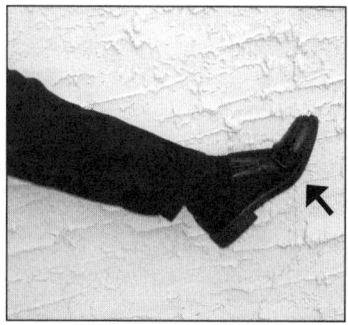

STRIKING WITH THE BALL OF FOOT

Instep Attack

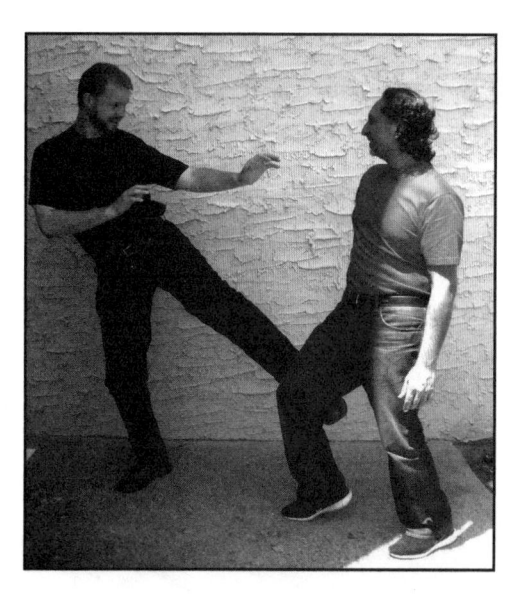

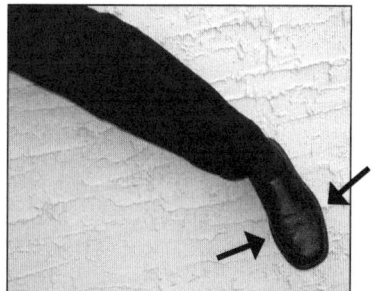

STRIKING WITH THE INSTEP

FOOT AND LEG ATTACKS

Full Foot Bottom

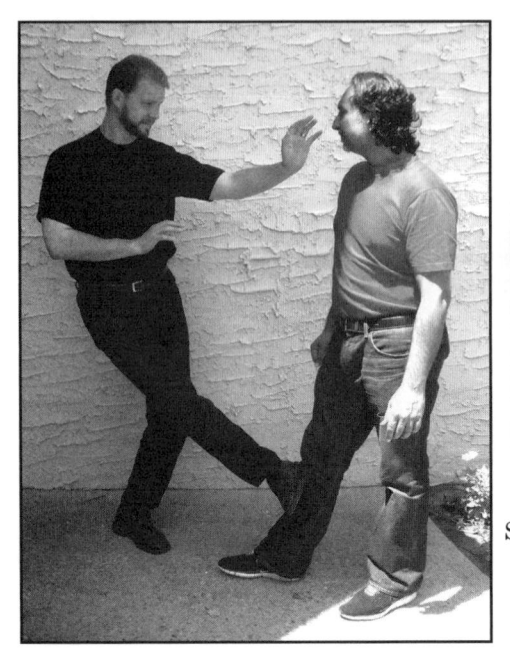

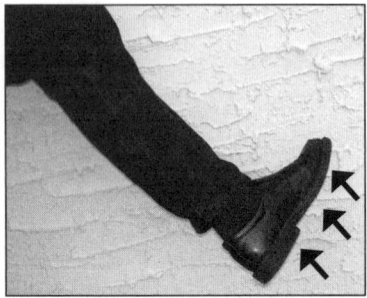

Striking with the full foot bottom

Kicks

Frontal kicks are swift, strong, and allow for the maintenance of balance. For the most part, the worst case scenario during a front kick is that your opponent blocks the attack and you have to reset yourself back into a safe stance. The basic front kick is defined by upward pointed toes, but make certain that it is the bottom of your foot that strikes the target. Consider as well that raising the foot too high can upset your center and allow your assailant to draw you into unsafe positioning.

Front Kick

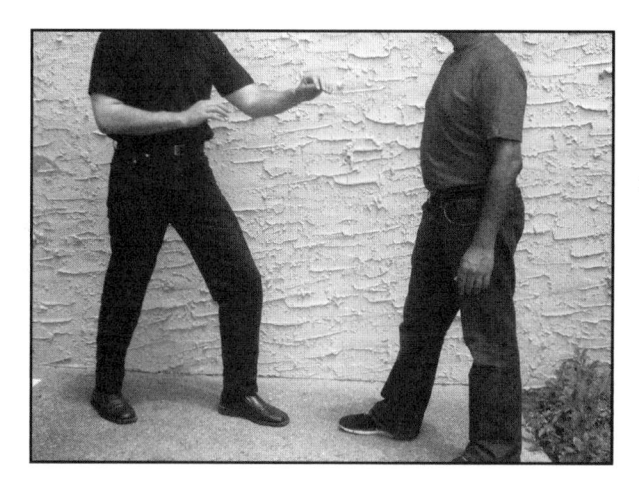

1. STANDING AT READY POSITION.

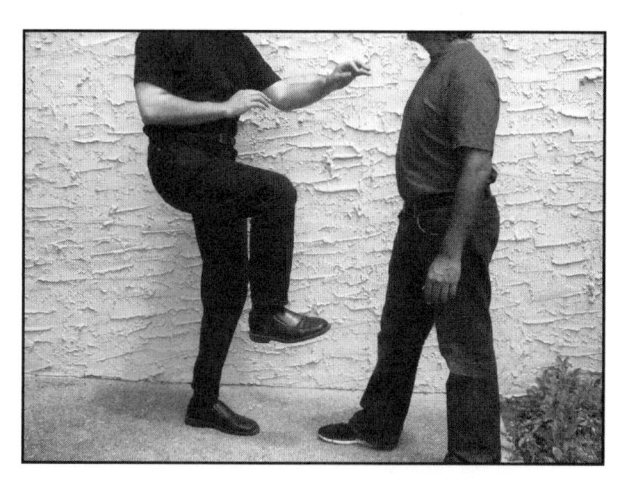

2. RAISE YOUR KICKING LEG AT THE KNEE.

FOOT AND LEG ATTACKS

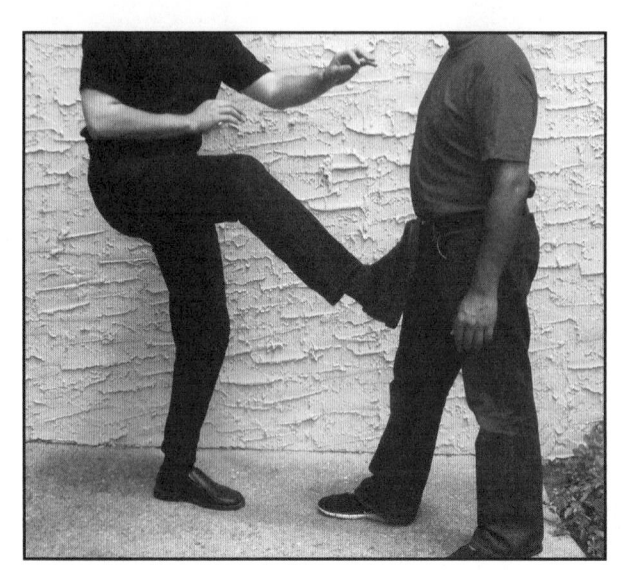

3. Press the bottom of your foot forward against the opponent.

Check Kick

Low kicks offer devastating power with little to no risk. Using the full bottom of your foot, better known as a "check kick," as the finish of a front kick (see below) and you will find one of the most, if not the safest kick ever devised.

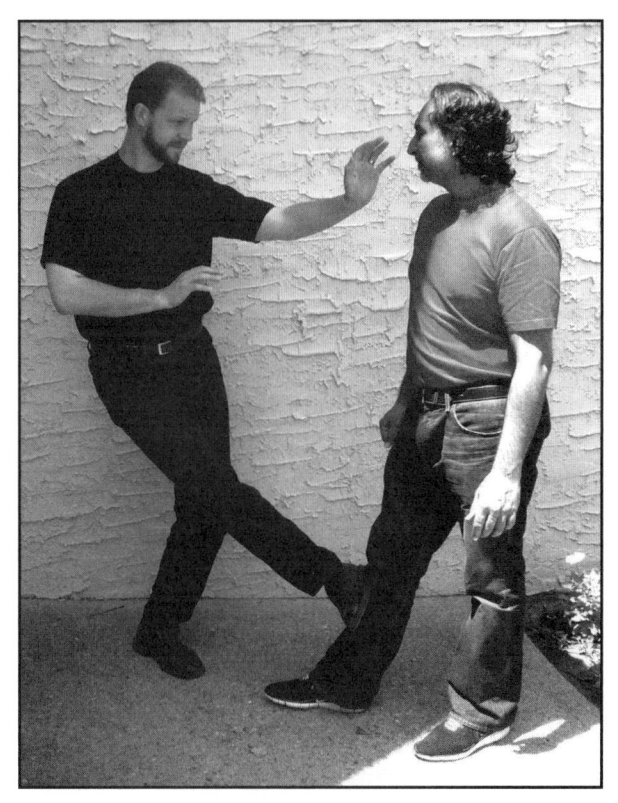

CHECK KICK - PRESS BOTTOM OF FOOT ONTO OPPONENT'S SHIN.

Back Kick

It is not uncommon for an experienced opponent to make his way behind you. If you find yourself facing the wrong way with your attacker clearly at your back, a back kick allows you the distance you will need to safely resume your readiness.

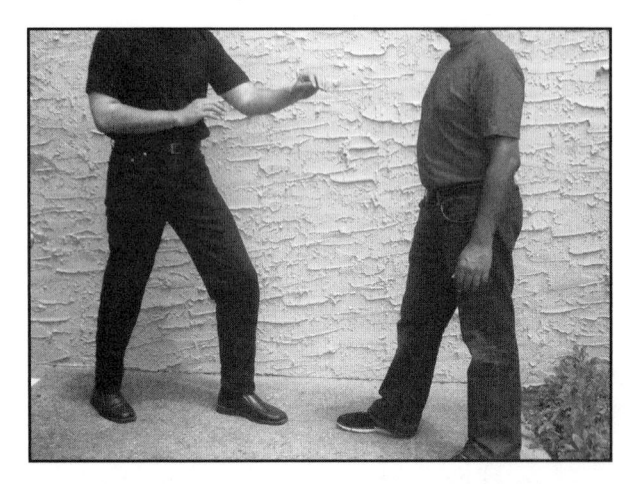

1. Standing at ready position.

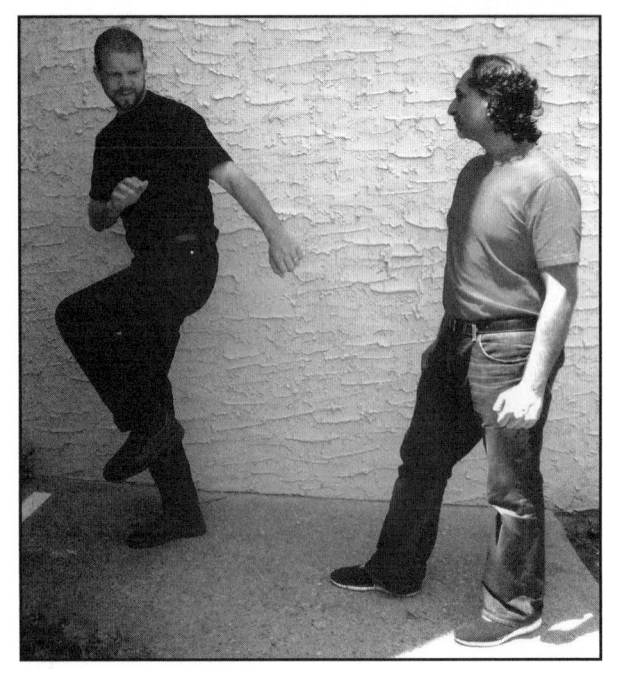

2. Turning yourself slightly to the side, lift your knee forward.

FOOT AND LEG ATTACKS

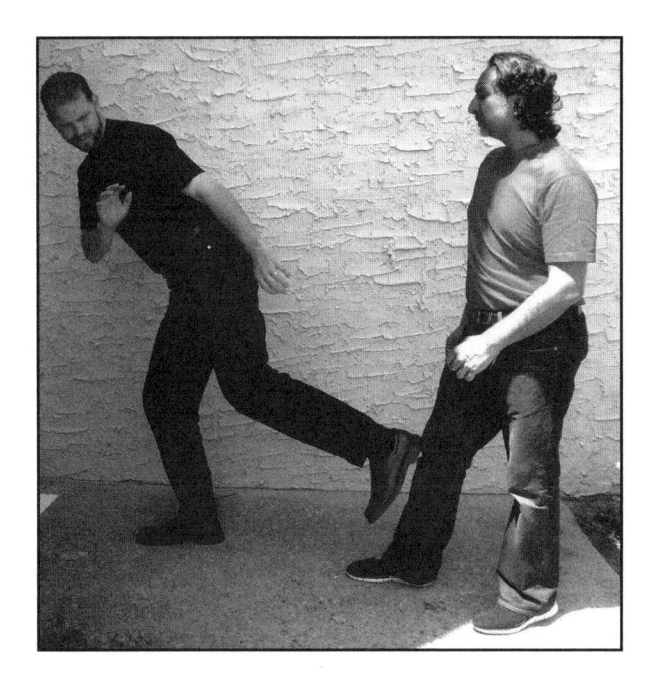

3. Aiming low behind yourself, slam bottom of the foot into the opponent's thigh, knee, or shin.

Side Kick

The side kick is commonly used during diamond fighting, but is by no means exclusive to this. The idea that every fight will be "one-on-one" is pleasant, but foolish. In the event of multiple attackers, side kicks can be a life saver.

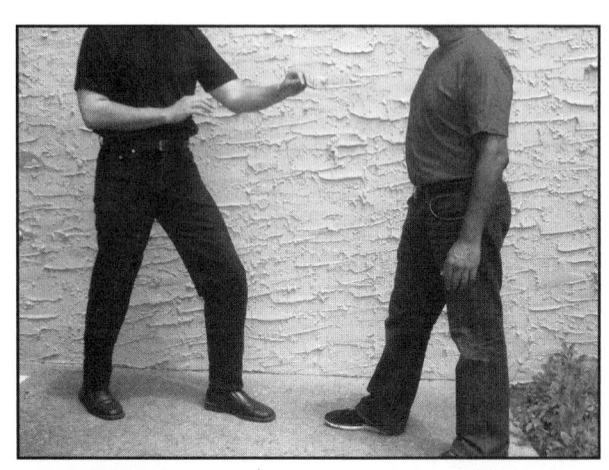

1. STANDING AT READY POSITION.

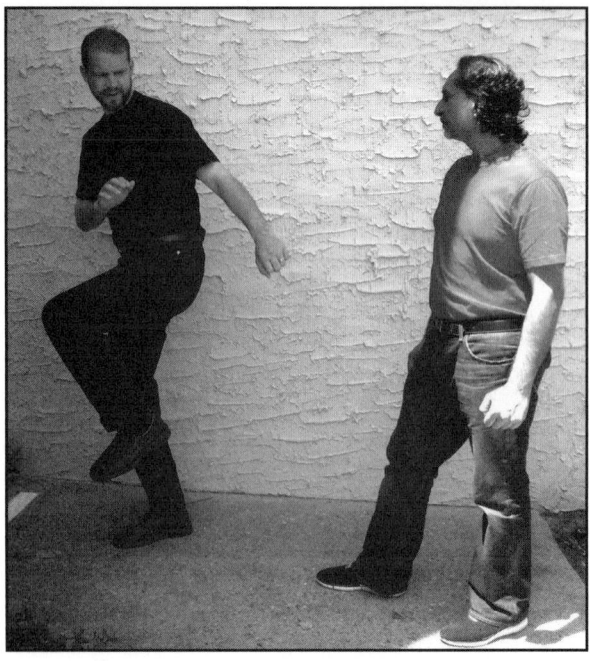

2. TURNING YOURSELF SLIGHTLY TO THE SIDE, LIFT YOUR KNEE FORWARD.

FOOT AND LEG ATTACKS

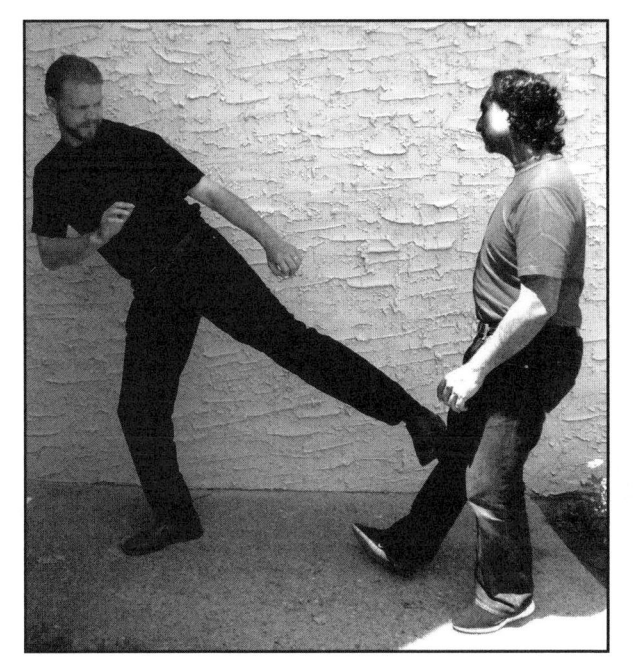

3. Aiming low to your side, slam the bottom of your foot into the opponent's thigh, knee, shin, or ankle.

Knee Attacks

Close quarter combat does not always allow for the bottom of the foot to be utilized. In the event of grappling, tunneling, or if you just find in-close fighting to be your preference, knee attacks allow for an amazing amount of strength with very little space for counter attack preparation.

When attempting any knee attack, remember to only strike with the top of the knee. Using the area below the kneecap allows for the possibility of severe personal damage including, but not limited to, dislocation.

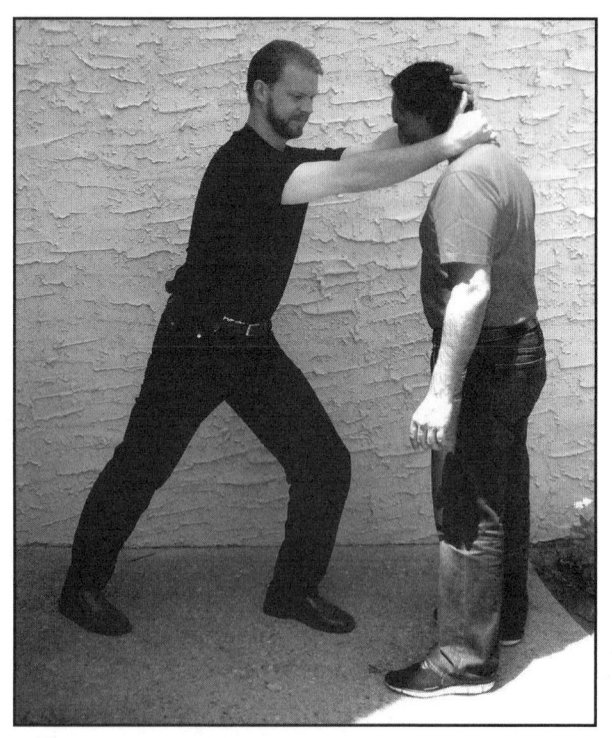

High-Level Knee Attack (Offensive)

1. FIRMLY GRAB THE OPPONENT AT THE BASE OF THE SKULL.

FOOT AND LEG ATTACKS

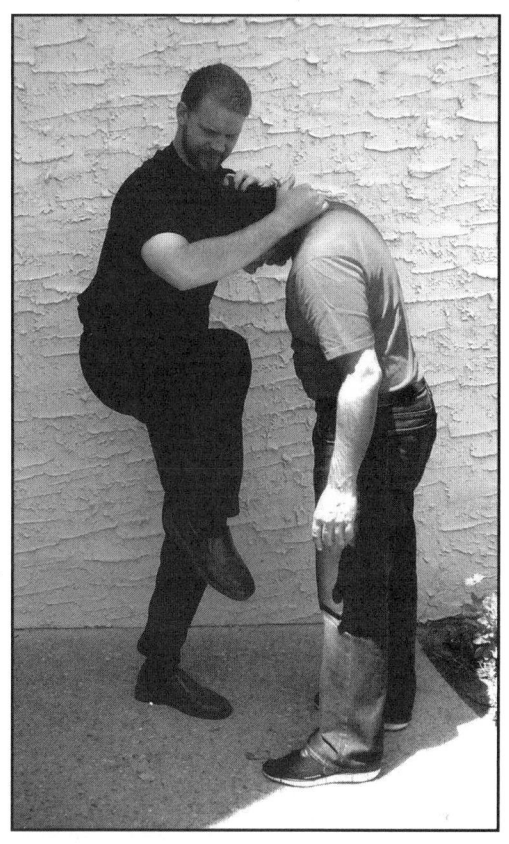

2. Turn slightly to one side while raising your knee to the desired target. Turning allows the opponent's energy to move past you instead of directly into you. This simple twist will permit greater stability and balance.

Low-Level Knee Attack (Offensive)

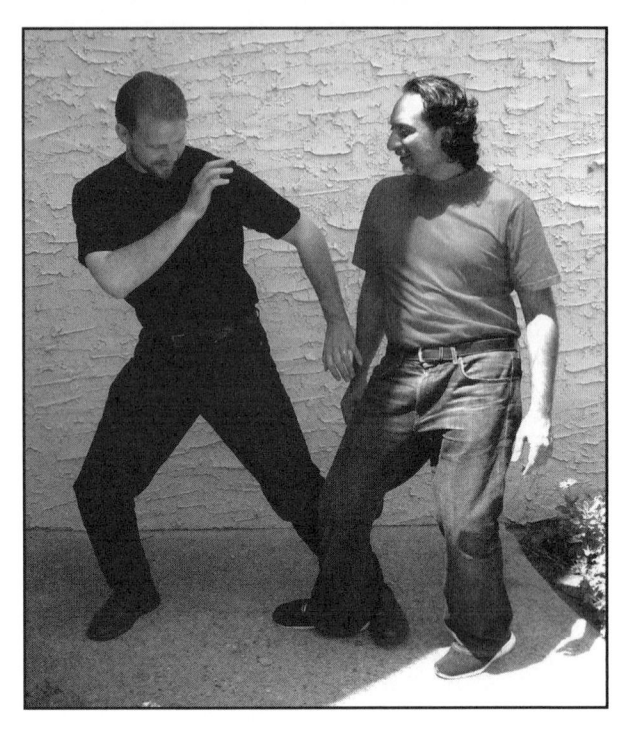

Taking a long step into your opponent's mirror leg, slam the top of your knee against his. This strike will pin your attacker's positioning if not land a devastating blow by itself.

CHAPTER 5
LOWER BODY DEFENSE

Defending oneself from kicks can be a totally safe practice. I say "can" because all too many times I have seen what should have been an easy block turn into a gross tactical error.

Legs are stronger than arms; no reasonable person will debate this fact. Taking a punch is one thing, but absorbing the raw power of a kick could easily end the fight before it has a chance to begin. There are several time proven methods to deflect, disarm, and diminish the strength of a kick. The purpose of the second part of this chapter is simply that, the complete avoidance of accepting such a devastating blow from your opponent. Lower body attacks create several difficult advantages such as power, speed, & distance, but they steal one vital component of our victory plan: balance.

Not once during my time as a bouncer did a fighter first attack me with a kick. Lower body attacks are rarely considered first by attackers, but this does not alter the fact that bouncers are always on the lookout for them. It is well known by any experienced member of a security team not only how destructive a kick can be, but how easy they are to defend against. When kicks are involved, any fight can easily be turned with just one block or even by simply walking forward at your attacker before their kick has a chance to peak.

There is another, flip side to this cautionary advise. A fight is easily lost to a skilled kicker by using improper blocking techniques. Such was the case with a rather large and rowdy drunk one night at "The Playroom." The man was grossly muscle bound to say the least and the very idea of having him get a hold on me was less than appetizing. Our hands met only for a few seconds before I threw my first kick to his shin. The joy of landing the kick was second only to my surprise in watching this behemoth dropping himself at the waist to block me instead of bending his knees. The human body is equipped with a large system of hinges called joints and no matter how many we have, most people seem to only rely on those above their waist to block kicks. With no more time needed to analyze this assailant, I proceeded to throw another fake kick low, drawing him once again into bending at his midsection. The very second before he attempted to grab onto my leg, I pulled it back and threw a hammer fist on the back of his head, ending the altercation. Had this fighter used common sense instead of flawed practice, the exchange might have ended very differently.

As simple as it seems to deflect your attackers foot from hitting you, injury often occurs from lack of proper technique. Absorbing the strength of a full kick can be tricky at best and painful at worst.

To simplify these lower body attacks, kicks are organized into 3 separate but equal blocking areas: High Level, Mid Level, and Low Level. Any one of these attacks can be attempted against you straight forward or from the side. For the benefit of the reader, both styles of attack will be covered for each level (where applicable.)

High Level Leg Attacks

Only persons believing their fighting skill to be much greater than it actually is will ever attempt a high kick in a real fight. Besides the fact that they take the most time to reach their target, they create new areas of possible injury. I have seen professionals land them quite accurately in the ring and instructors connect with ease when on the mats, but the real world offers much less hope of successfully achieving this brand of attack. As you will see, defense against this style of kick is very simple and whether the attack comes straight forward at you or from the side, the defense is the same.

High-Level Kick (Defensive)

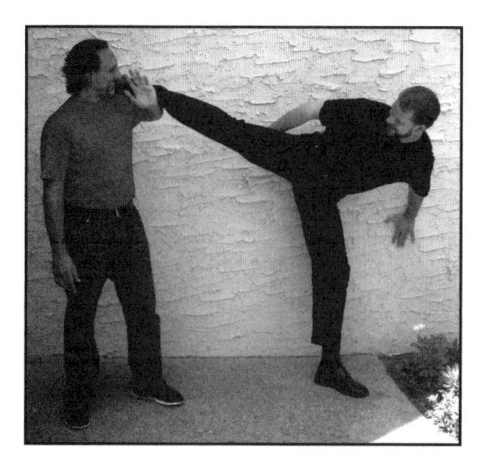

1. USING A SIMPLE UPWARD BLOCKING ARM WITH AND OUTWARD BENT WRIST, DEFLECT THE UNDERSIDE OF THE ANKLE.

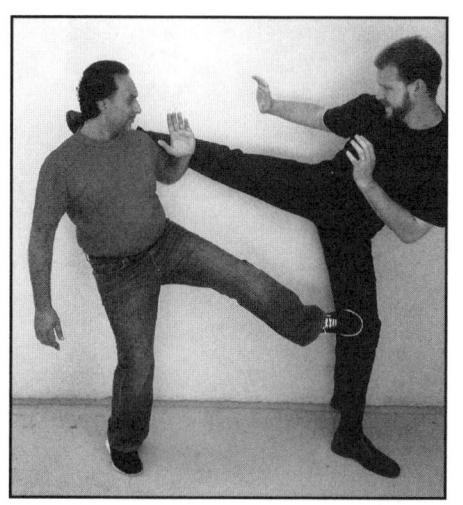

2. BEFORE YOUR ATTACKER HAS A CHANCE TO RECOIL HIS LEG, THROW A SIDE KICK TO THE KNEE OF HIS STANDING LEG.

LOWER BODY DEFENSE

There is another type of kick that an opponent may attempt during a confrontation and it deserves a special mention. If your assailant is foolish enough to throw a flying kick, count yourself as lucky, accept the gift of their ignorance, and proceed with the following steps.

1. For a flying spin kick, take one large step forward.

2. For any kind of forward jumping kick, take one large step to the side.

Yep, that's it. That's how simple defeating a flying kick is. Take one large step either way and you have defeated the strike. Here is the explanation: When an attacker lofts themselves upward and spins, they have stolen any balance they might have maintained had they remained on the ground. Once they have jumped up, it is impossible to alter their flight pattern. In other words, they can't recognize that their target has moved forward, correct the mistake by flying backwards, reset the point of impact, and then land the kick. Instead, what will happen is the attack (Mid-thigh at it's new point of impact) will land harmlessly upon your blocking arm. After this the attacker will plummet to the ground accepting all of the force of the fall.

As for straight forward jump kick: Let the attacker waste precious energy and tire himself out by throwing himself upward time and time again. You will have ample chance to injure the assailant after his descent, if he hasen't already done it himself.

Mid-Level Leg Attacks

Accepting the power of a leg strike into the stomach or ribcage is an excruciating thing. Mid-level attacks take less time to land than a high kick, but offer the same devastation with half of the risk. The best advice to prevent your assailant from landing a mid-level attack is to stand properly (in the Ward-Off Position). Keeping your hands in front of you will grant the opportunity to deflect most of the blocks and dissuade most of the attempts. Grabbing & pulling may be used for mid-level attacks whether straight forward or side attacks if you can catch the assailant's foot. Either result can create the opportunity to effectively fall your opponent with little difficulty. Should your opponent attack in this manner, the following tactics may be employed:

Mid-Level Attack (Mirror)

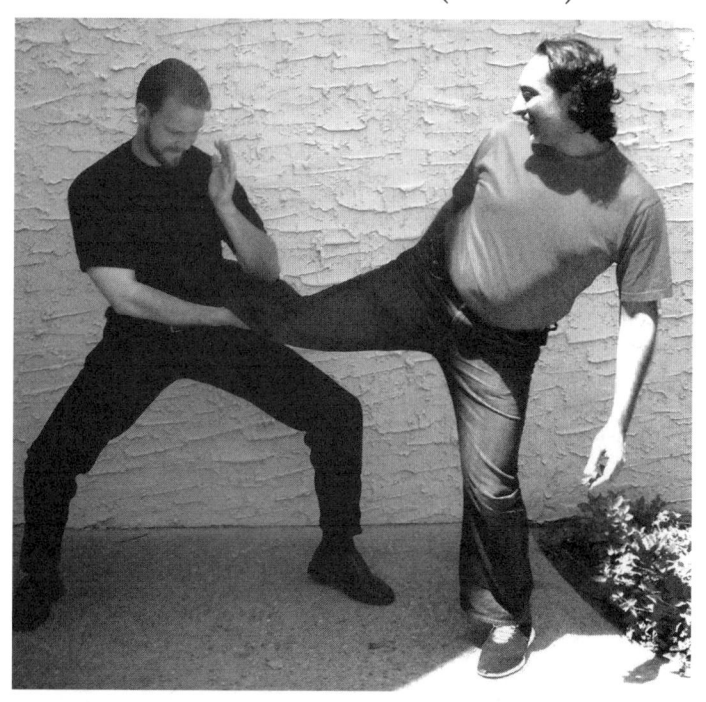

Keeping your elbows at your sides, bend your knees and twist your hips to defend. Drop your elbow directly into opponent's attack.

LOWER BODY DEFENSE

Mid-Level Attack Side (Cross)

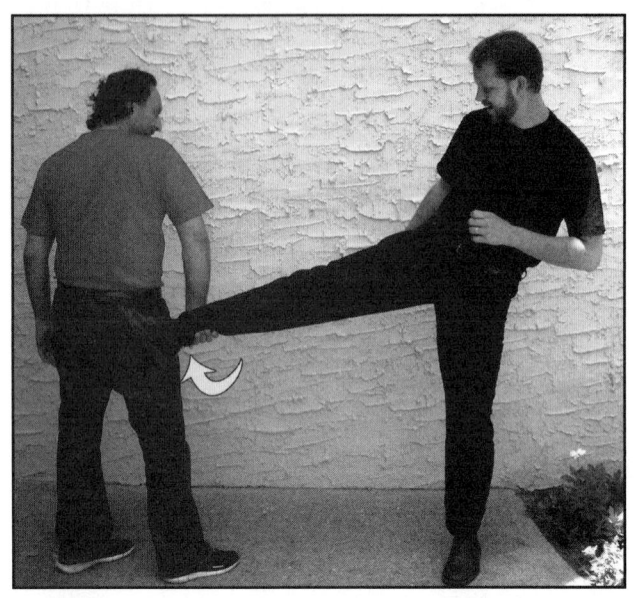

1. Use a downward block to grab your attacker's kick and press it outward and away from your body.

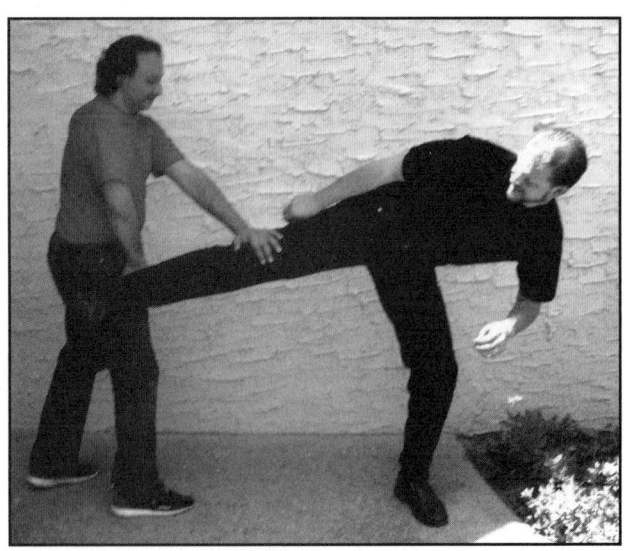

2. Turning yourself back toward your attacker, press downward atop the side of their knee.

LOWER BODY DEFENSE

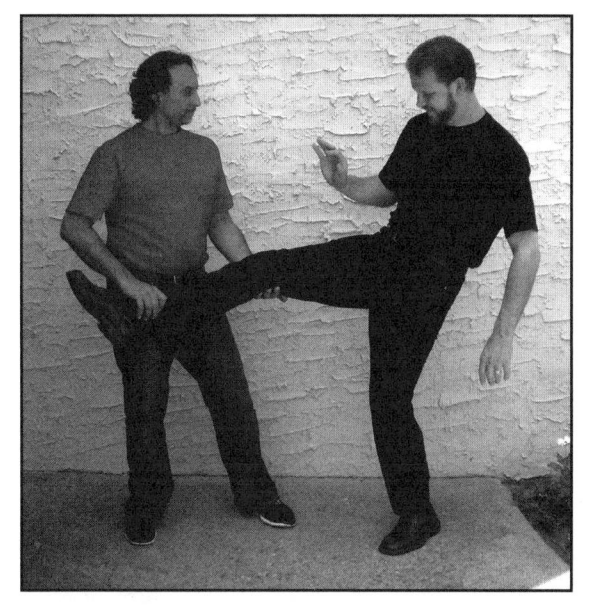

3. (OPTIONAL) CONTINUE BY PULLING OPPONENT TOWARD YOU.

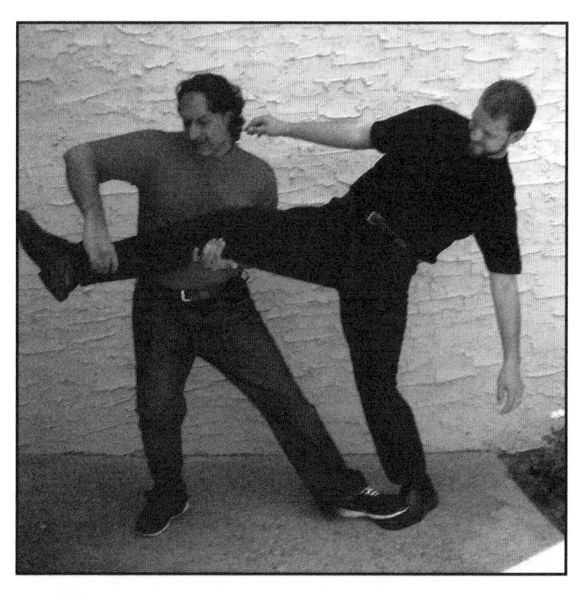

4. (OPTIONAL) PLACE YOUR CROSS FOOT OVER THEIR STANDING LEG AND PULL.

LOWER BODY DEFENSE

Mid-Level Attack Forward

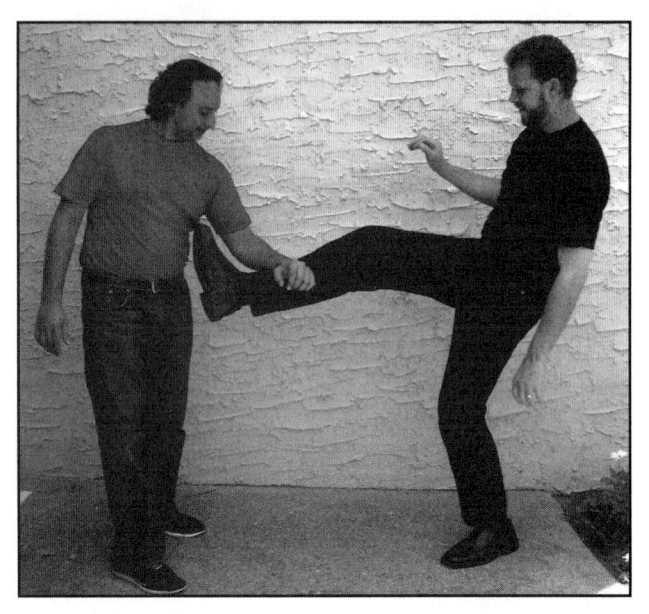

1. BLOCK THE TOP OF THE KICK DOWNWARD WITH YOUR WRIST/FOREARM.

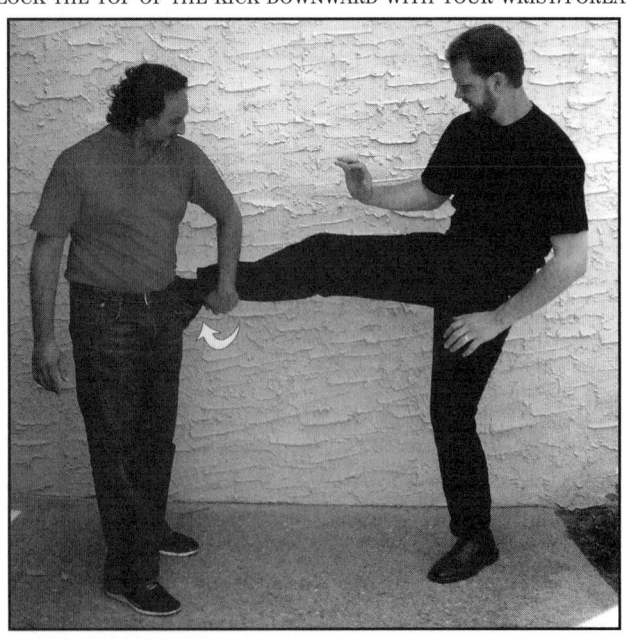

2. DEFLECT THE KICK BY SCOOPING IT OUTSIDE AND AWAY FROM YOUR BODY.

LOWER BODY DEFENSE

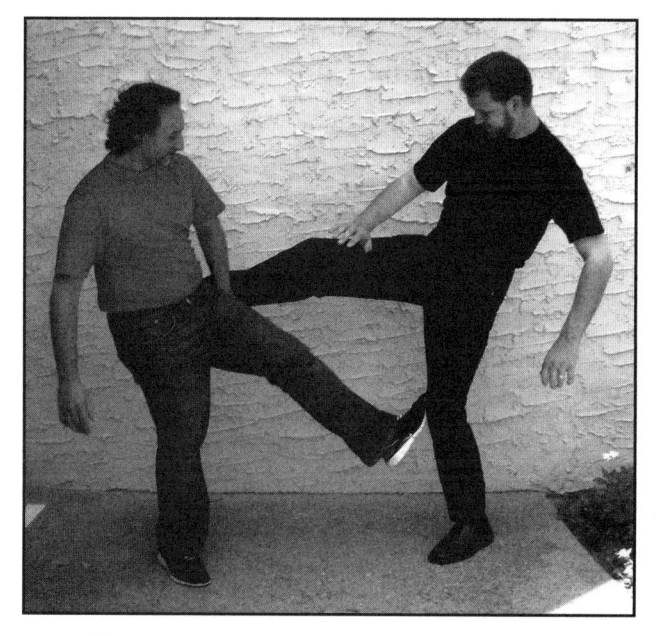

3. Level a kick on the inside of attacker's knee.

Recommended Finishing Strikes: Side Kick, Instep

Knee Attack (Defensive)

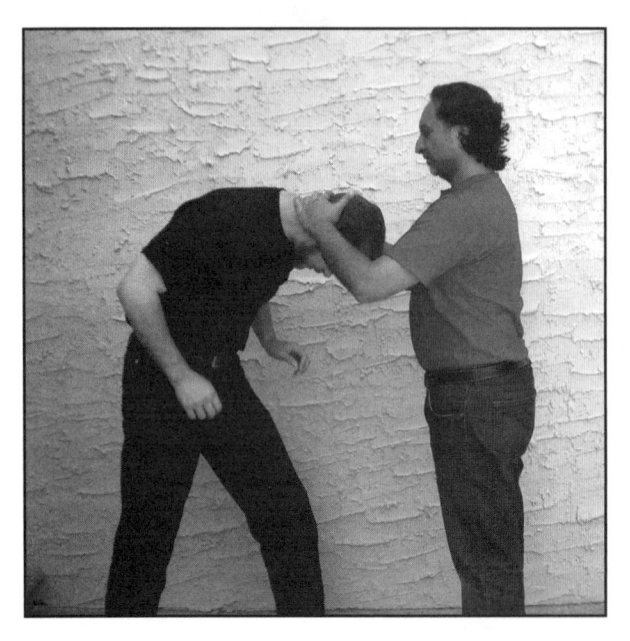

1. The attacker grabs back of your head.

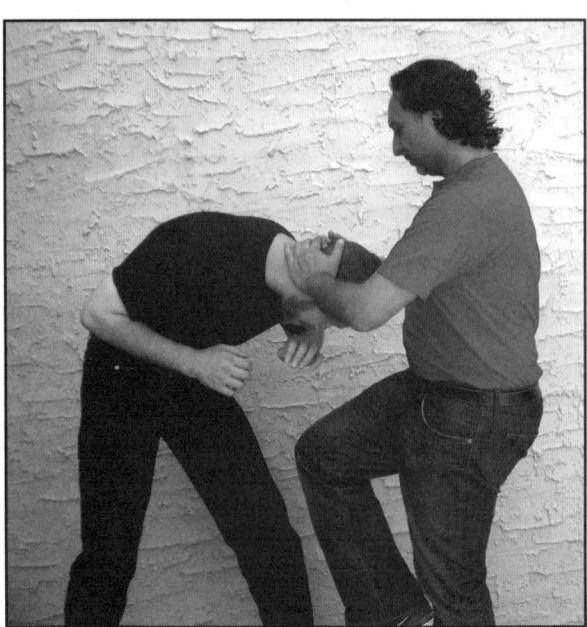

2. Prep your mirror hand as the attacker lifts his knee for an attack.

LOWER BODY DEFENSE

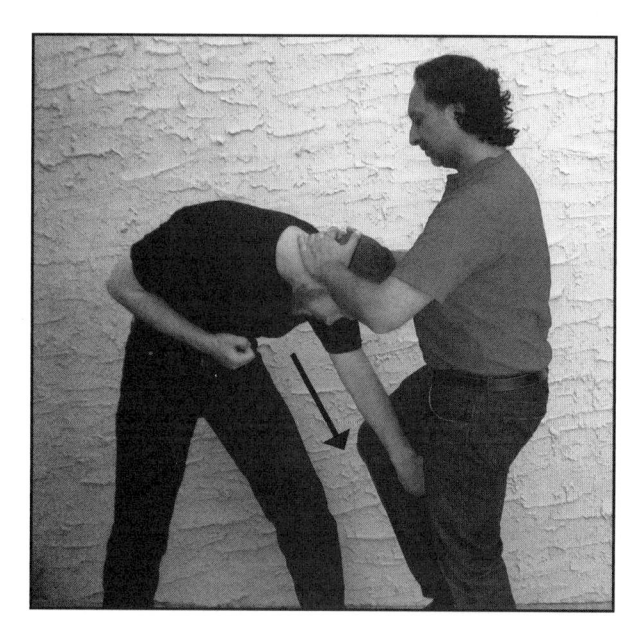

3. PUNCH DOWNWARD BETWEEN THE OPPONENT'S LEGS, GRAZING THE INSIDE OF THE ATTACKING KNEE WITH YOUR WRIST AND FOREARM.

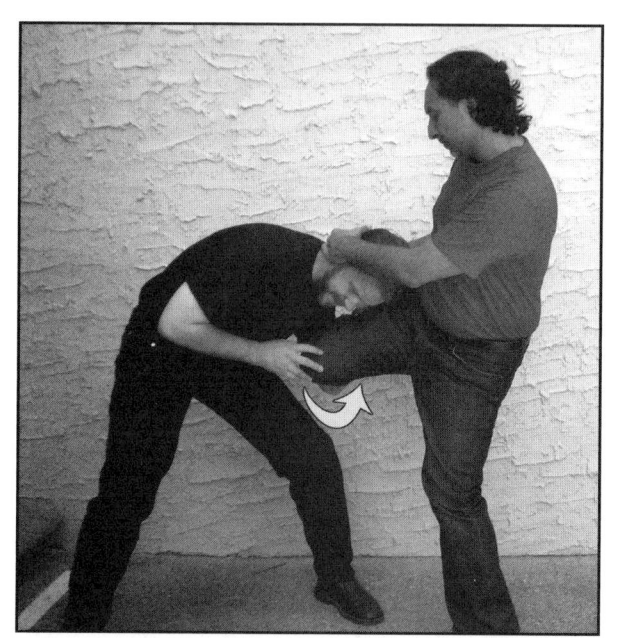

4. HOOK YOUR ARM UNDERNEATH AND AROUND THE OUTSIDE OF THE ATTACKING LEG.

LOWER BODY DEFENSE

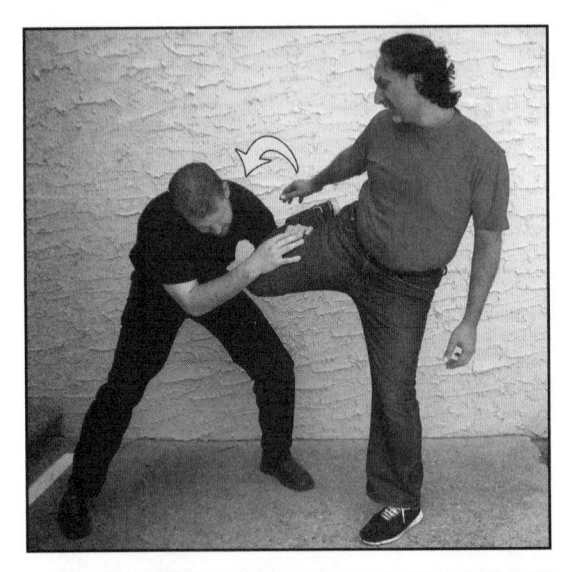

5. CIRCLE YOUR ARM COMPLETELY AROUND THE ATTACKER'S LEG AND PRESS DOWNWARD ON THE INSIDE OF THE KNEE.

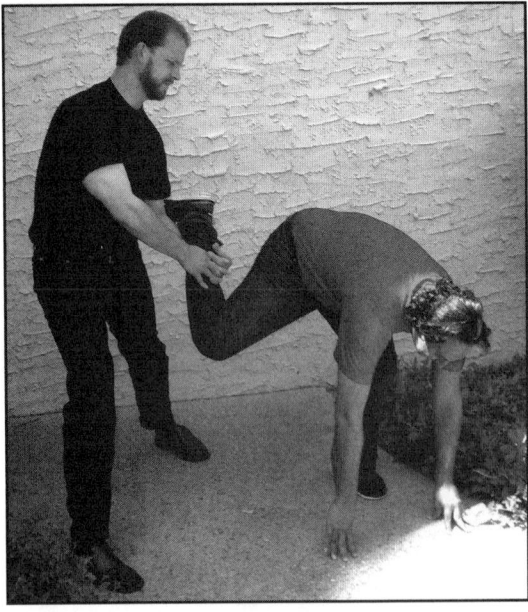

6. CONTINUE THIS MOVEMENT UNTIL THE LEVER ACTION ON THE KNEE CAUSES YOUR OPPONENT TO FALL.

Important Safety Note: To avoid injury always move the force of a mid level leg attack to your side. Do not attempt to absorb the strength of any kick or knee by striking at it with you hand or palm! More than fingers may be broken.

Low Level Leg Attacks

Having previously stated that low kicks are among the safest and most practical of all kicking techniques, it is almost assured that any experienced fighter will attempt these attacks. The best manner in which to block these offenses is by altering a simple check kick to a defensive tactic. The bottom of each of your feet absorbs thousands of pounds every day just by standing and walking. By using the underside of your foot, you can withstand the pressure of even the strongest attack. Adding a few more pounds per square inch does very little damage if accepted properly. Regardless of the type of kick attempted by your assailant, check kicks will choke any low attack without turning you from your opponent

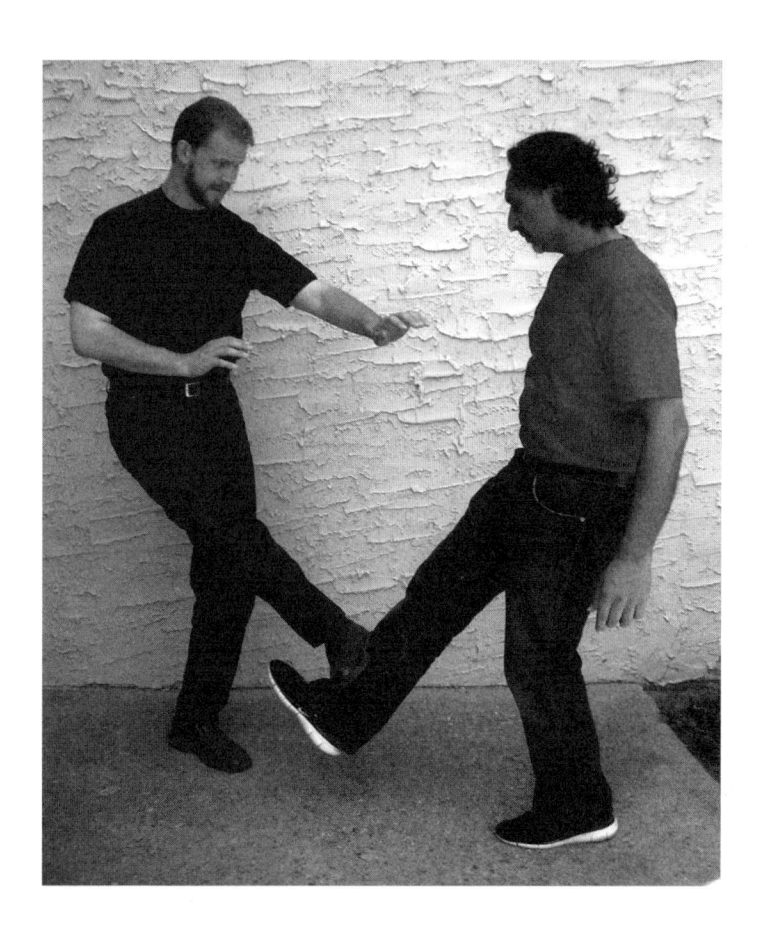

CHAPTER 6
LOCKS, GRAPPLING and FREEING

Grappling is a common and undeniable part of most fights. There are several variations and types of grappling, but one thing is constant: close quarter combat.

Bouncers are trained to use grappling and holds for most of their job. The reason is more than just simply wanting to avoid giving a patron a bloody nose and damaging the reputation of the club. Locking someone into submission creates a mindset of their own lacking control and, hopefully, reduces their desire to continue fighting.

In one instance at "The Gate," I found myself face to face with an aggressive, semi-professional boxer. The customer had been drinking heavily and bragging all night that he knocked people out for a living. Arrogance is one thing, but when pride is fueled by alcohol, trouble is brewing. It was only a matter of time before this drunkard started a skirmish. On my arrival to the fight, I witnessed this attacker knock his opponent down with one strike. Knowing that I wanted no part of his expertly trained knuckles, I took to mind only those moves which would keep them from me. After deflecting a single punch, I threw myself inward at him, clutching my forearms across his chest and neck and twisting him to the ground with myself on top. In less than a second, he physically and verbally submitted to my hold. I had no intention of trying to match this assailant at his own game and considered the fear he would feel in being taken down so quickly and decisively. I knew that if I could throw him off guard for even one second, that I would have the fight.

To illuminate the best possible techniques for each situation, the locks and grappling techniques have been separated into parts. Each section will describe and prepare you for the most common possibilities.

Headlocks

Taking control of someone's head will all but render them useless. Options include loss of oxygen and unconsciousness, not to mention the grave danger of injury to the vertebrae and spine. This is no alarm if we are on the giving end of the lock, but consider the alternate possibility. Understandably now, freeing ourselves from headlocks will be our first priority.

Forward Facing Headlock (Defensive)

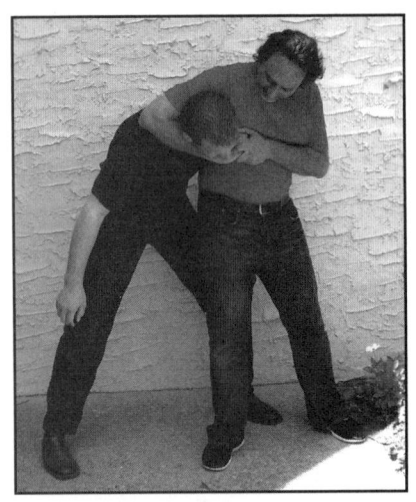

1. THE ATTACKER PLACES YOU IN A FORWARD-FACING HEADLOCK.

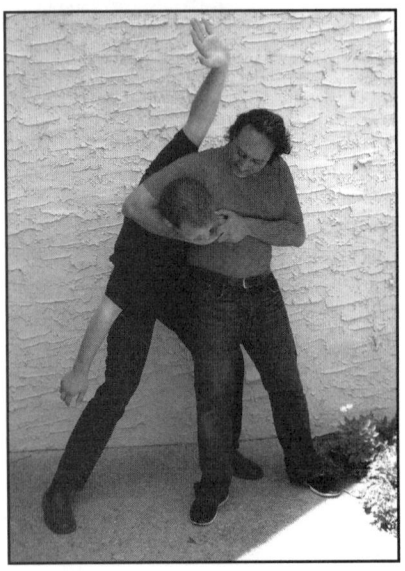

2. FROM BEHIND, LIFT THE HAND CLOSEST (THE NEAR/MIRROR HAND) TO YOUR ATTACKER.

LOCKS, GRAPPLING AND FREEING

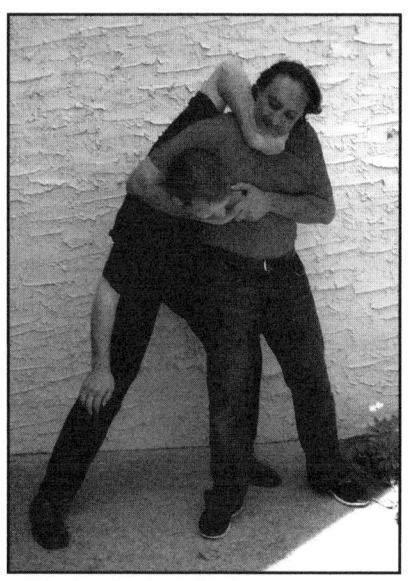

3. Reach your near/mirror hand over the shoulder that maintains the hold on you and place a Claw Hand attack at the opponent's throat.

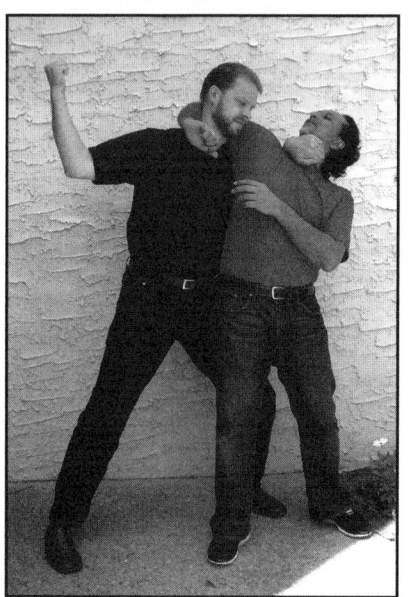

4. Pull back on the throat and stand up.

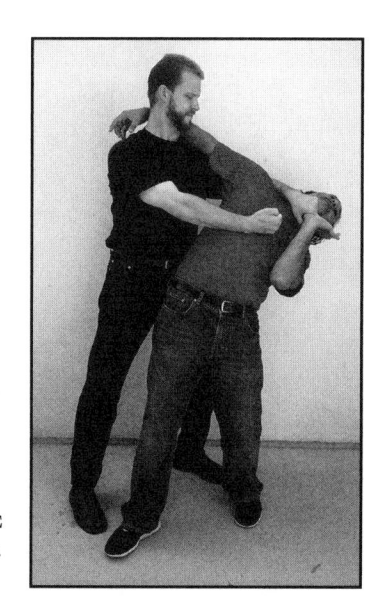

5. (Extra) Finish with a chop to the opponent's neck or heart.

Forward Facing Headlock (Offensive)

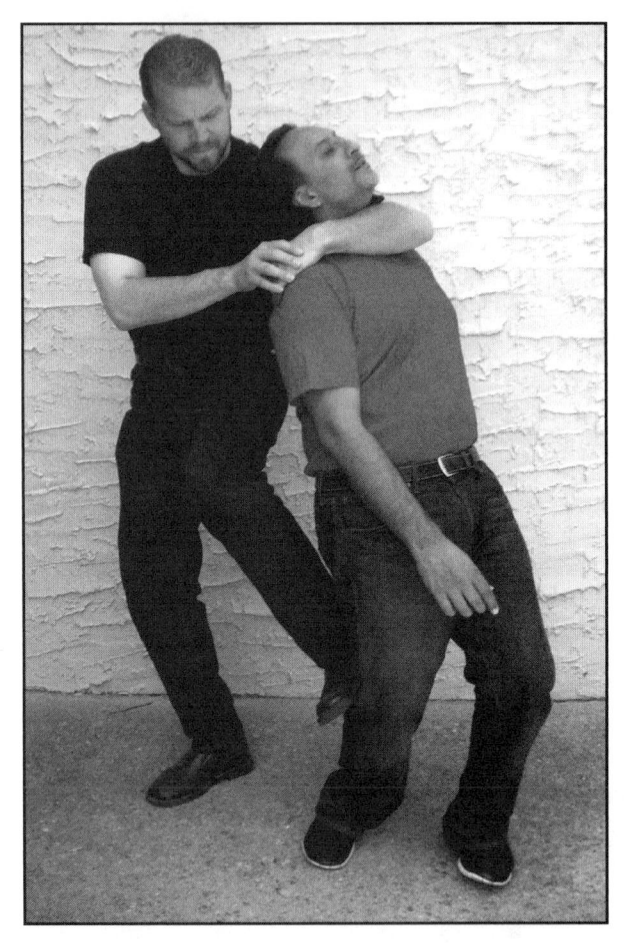

Place the inside of your elbow across the opponent's throat, grasping the wrist with your free hand. Make certain to press on the back of his knee with your foot so he cannot regain mobility. Turning to the side will add greatly to your stability.

LOCKS, GRAPPLING AND FREEING

Backward Facing Headlock (Defensive)

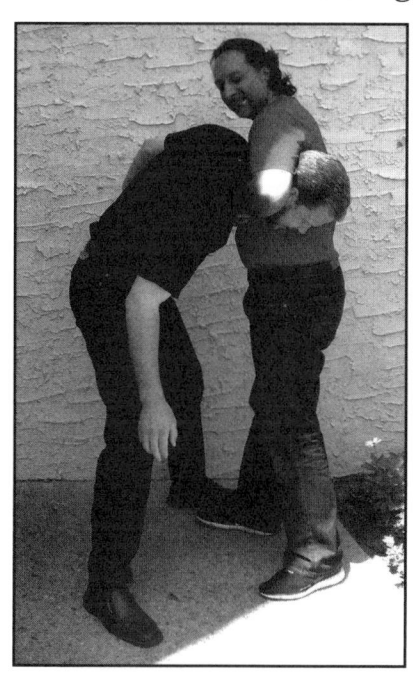

1. Reach your near/cross hand from your side and place your palm on the neck of the attacker.

2. Using your far/mirror hand, grab the inside of the knee.

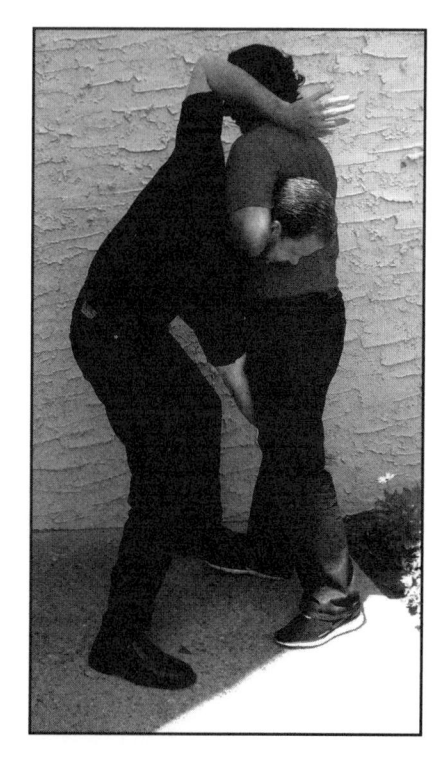

LOCKS, GRAPPLING AND FREEING

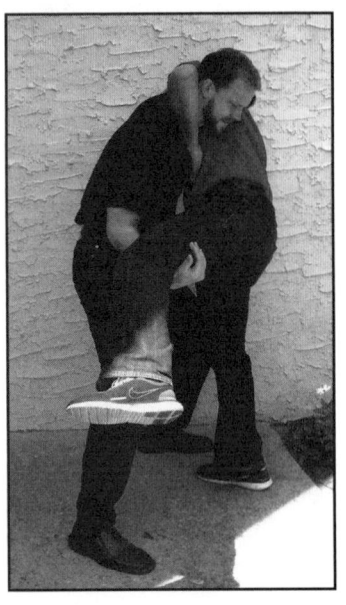

3. Pushing the head downward, lift the knee upward, spinning the opponent to the ground head first.

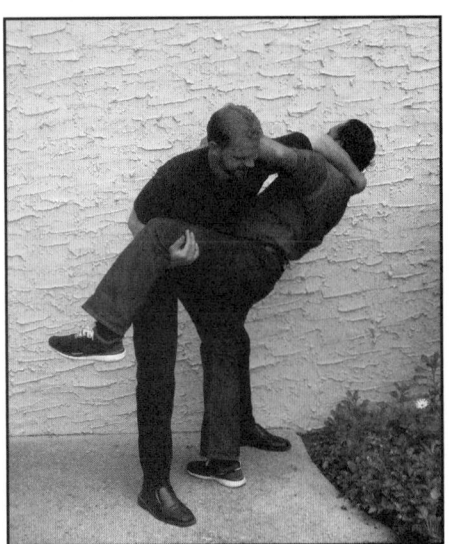

4. Take the opponent off balance by standing and tipping forward.

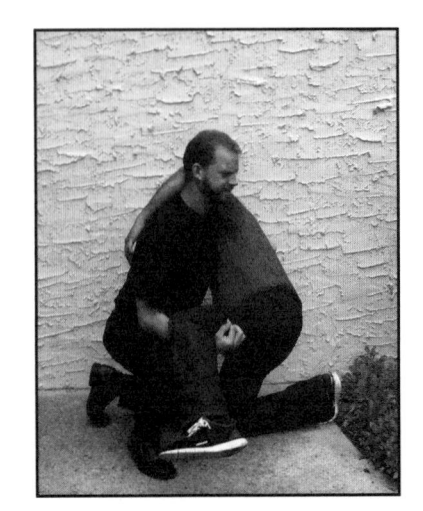

5. Kneel to finish the submission.

Backward Facing Headlock (Offensive)

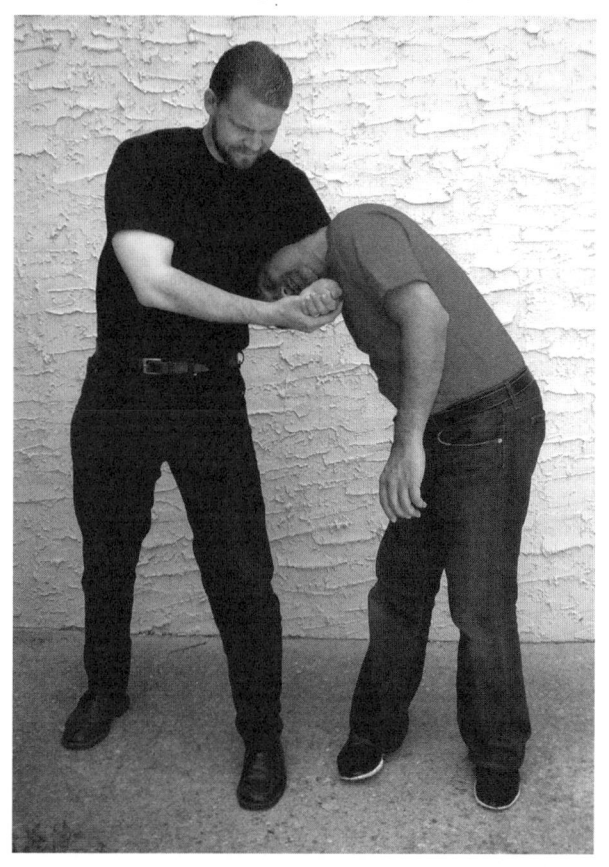

Maintain the headlock by cupping the attacker's chin on the inside of your wrist and twisting upward. Turning your body to the side will once again disable the attacker's ability to knock you over by pushing backward.

Full Nelson (Defensive)

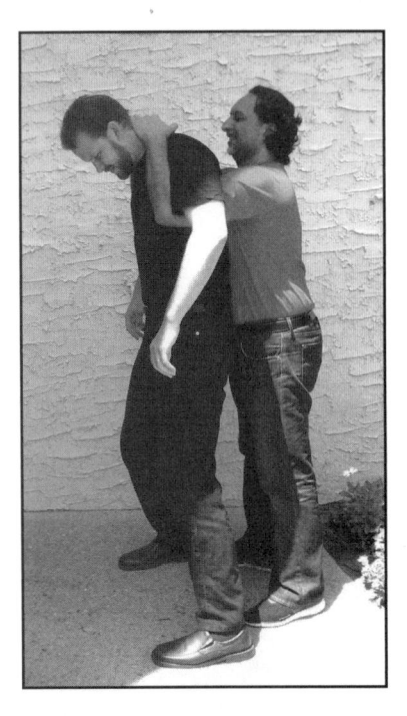

1. The attacker places you in a full nelson headlock.

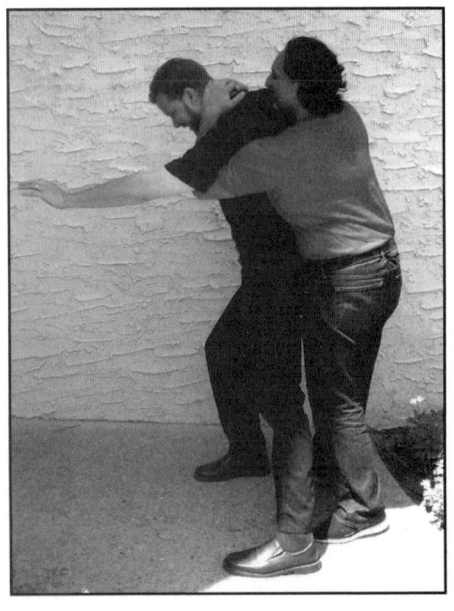

2. Throw your first hand forward in punching manner.

LOCKS, GRAPPLING AND FREEING

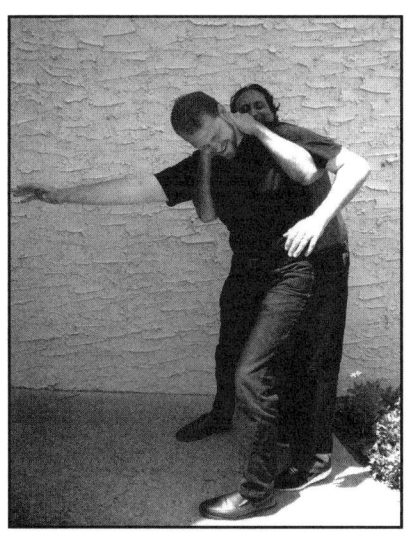

3. Continue repeated punching with your other arm.

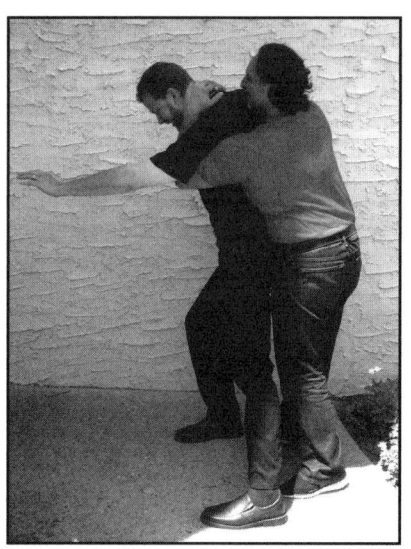

4. Repeat moves 2 & 3 over and over, each time weakening your attacker's hold.

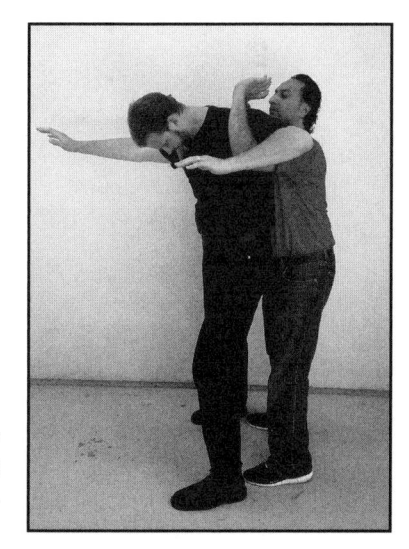

5. Eventually, the attacker's grip will loosen enough to free yourself from the hold.

LOCKS, GRAPPLING AND FREEING

Double Handed Choke (Defensive)

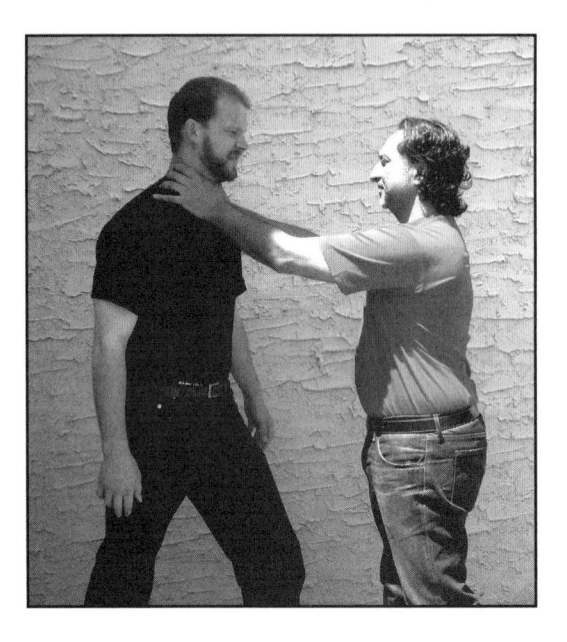

1. THE OPPONENT PLACES BOTH HANDS ON YOUR NECK.

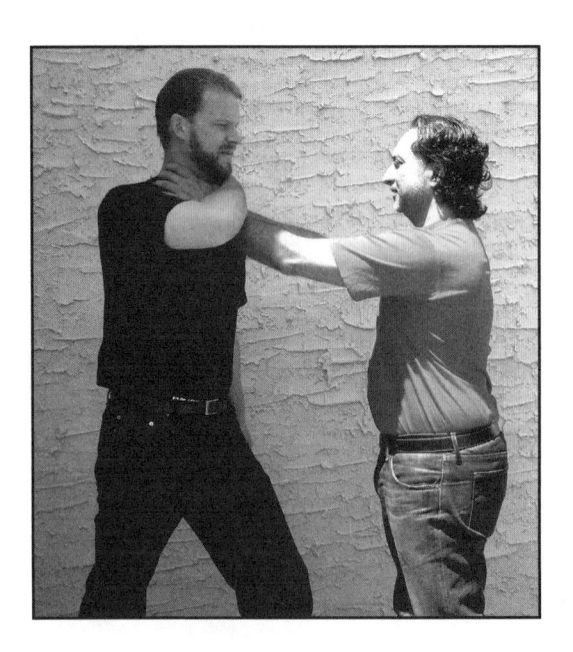

2. RAISING EITHER HAND, TIGHTLY COVER THE ATTACKING HANDS, PINNING THEM TO YOUR HIGH CHEST.

LOCKS, GRAPPLING AND FREEING

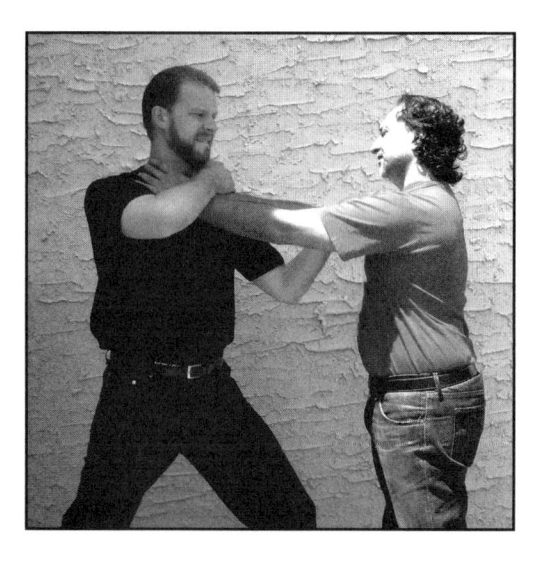

3. Use your free hand to strike upward between the gap in your attacker's arms.

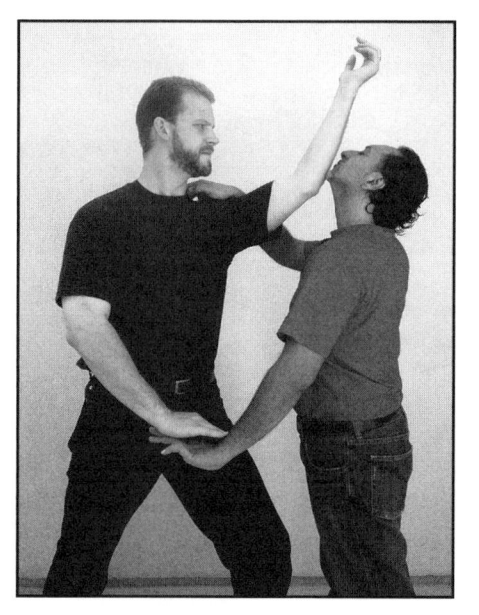

4. Pull the attacker's arm down from your neck while finishing with a blow to the face.

Recommended Finishing Strikes: Knife Hand, Obtuse Angle Elbow Strike, Acute Angle Elbow Strike

Body Locks

Body locks can be quite painful, but are rarely more than a slight inconvenience. Therefore, we will only refer to them in the defensive manner.

Bear Hug (Defensive)

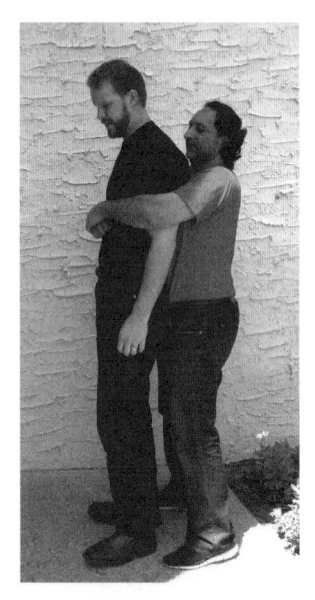

1. THE ATTACKER APPLIES A BEAR HUG.

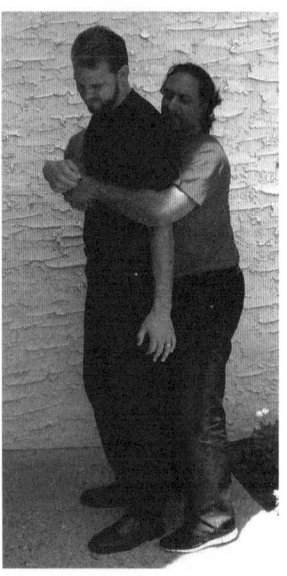

2. MAKE YOUR FREE HAND INTO A KNUCKLE RAKE OR STARFIST/EAGLE'S BEAK HAND. SLAM IT AGAINST THE MIDDLE OF THE ATTACKER'S TOP HAND.

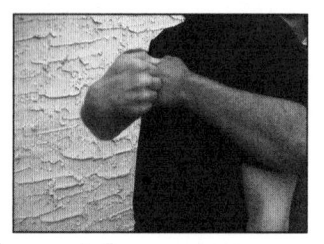

(CLOSE UP) IF YOUR FIRST ATTEMPT TO FREE YOURSELF FAILS, TRY, TRY AGAIN.

LOCKS, GRAPPLING AND FREEING

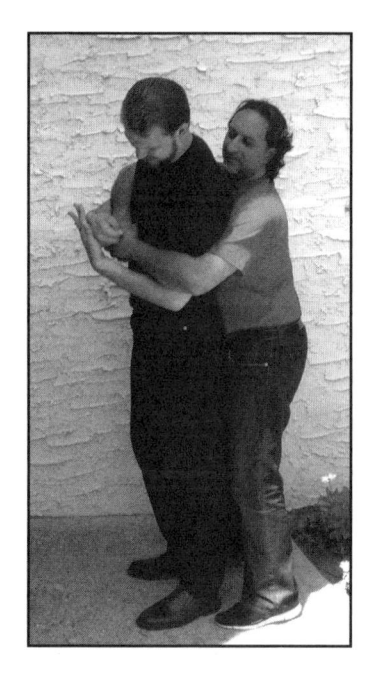

3. (OPTIONAL) IF MOBILITY PERMITS, USE YOUR FREE HAND TO SLAM OVER YOUR OWN FIST, LIKE A HAMMER HITTING A CHISEL.

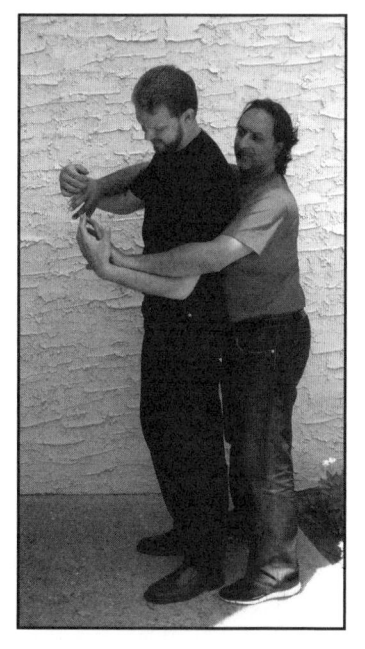

4. ONCE THE ATTACKER'S GRIP IS LOOSENED, USE BOTH HANDS TO PULL HIS WRISTS AWAY FROM YOU.

Wrist & Arm Locks

There are few things more painful than a broken wrist. Control of the entire body can be achieved from this location. Relieving pressure and removing the chance of injury are not difficult however. Following simple guidelines and understanding the possibilities and limitations of the human body, we can protect ourselves from harm.

Arm Bar (Defensive)

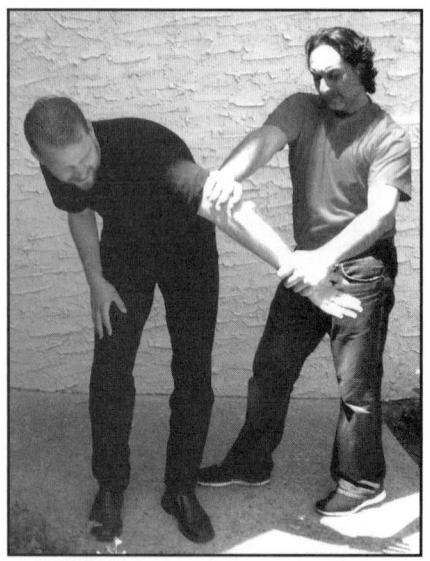

1. THE OPPONENT PLACES YOU IN AN ELBOW-LOCKED ARM BAR.

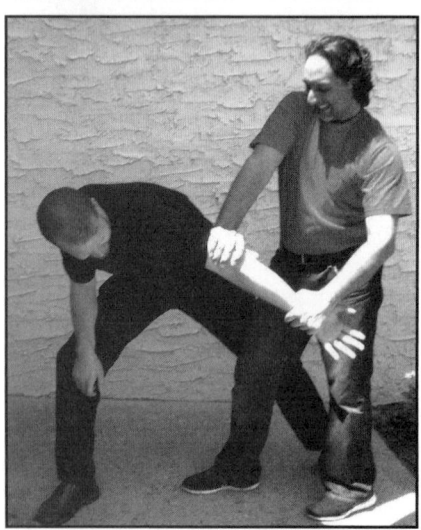

2. STEP BEHIND YOUR OPPONENT WITH YOUR NEAR LEG, MAKING FIRM CONTACT WITH THE BACK OF HIS KNEE(S).

LOCKS, GRAPPLING AND FREEING

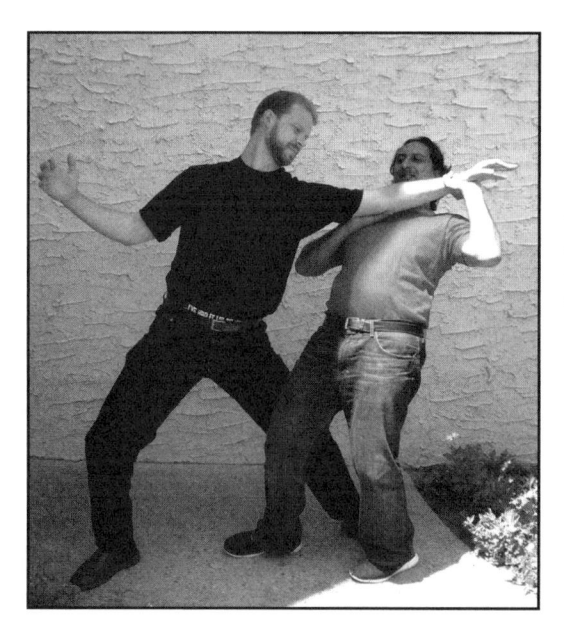

3. Press on the back of the opponent's knee and stand straight up. The pressure on the back of his leg(s) will take away his control.

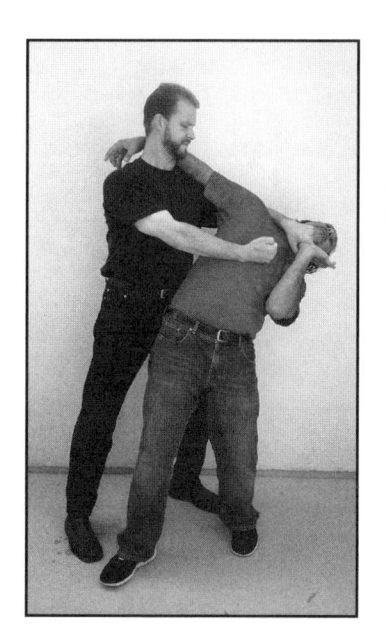

4. (Optional) Land a finishing chop once you take control.

Arm Bar (Offensive)

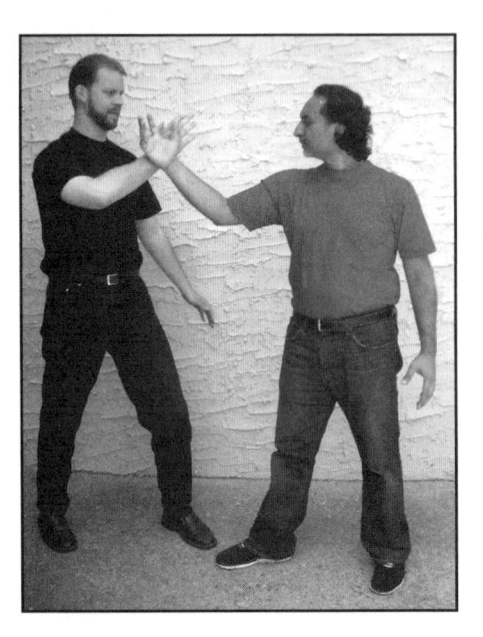

1. BLOCK THE OPPONENT'S ARM ON THE OUTSIDE OF HIS ATTACKING WRIST WITH YOUR CROSS HAND.

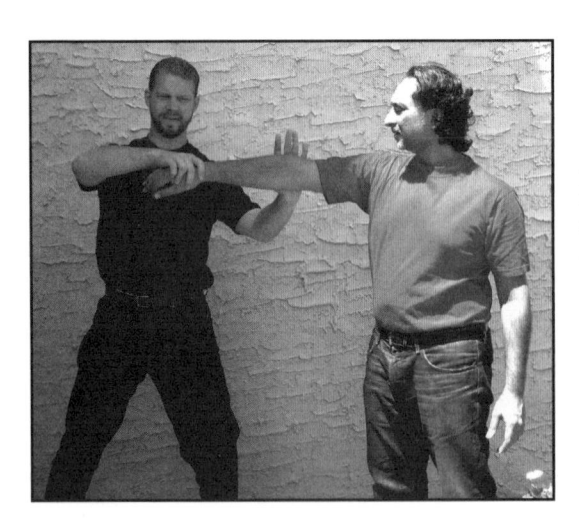

2. PULL THE OPPONENT'S ARM PAST YOURSELF AND ADD PRESSURE TO THE ELBOW OF THE ATTACKING ARM.

LOCKS, GRAPPLING AND FREEING

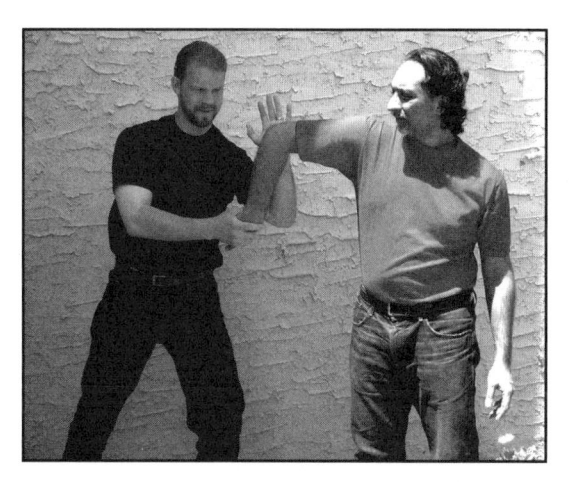

3. LOWER THE WRIST OF THE ATTACKING ARM AND CHANGE THE PRESSURE ON HIS ELBOW TO A TWISTING/TORQUE MOTION. KEEPING THE ELBOW STRAIGHT CAN AND USUALLY WILL ALLOW THE OPPONENT TO FREE HIMSELF.

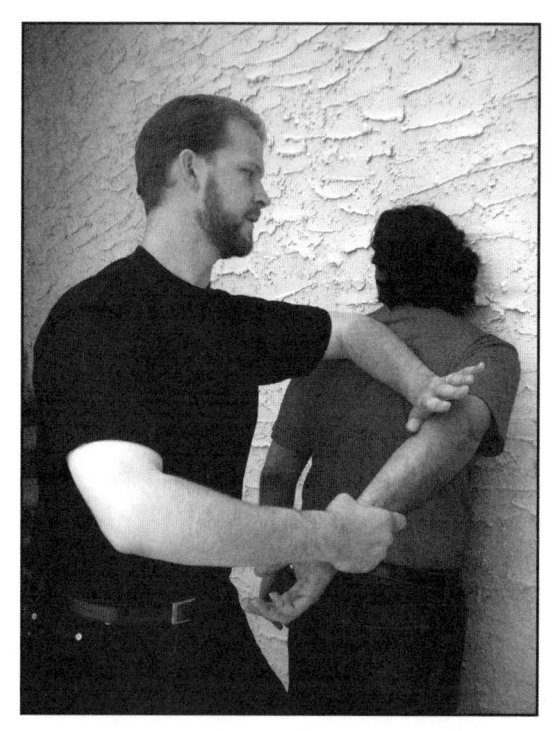

4. (OPTIONAL) USING A WALL OR EVEN THE GROUND, PRESS THE OPPONENT'S BODY FIRMLY AGAINST A BARRIER. THIS TECHNIQUE GREATLY LESSENS THE ABILITY YOUR ATTACKER TO FREE HIMSELF.

Wrist Grabs

There are two types of grabs, empty and full. Before any action is taken, the recognition of which grab has been applid by your opponent is a must. An empty grab is attained once contact and restraint are achieved, but no further manipulation is tried. A full grab is accomplished only during or upon completion of a full submission. With an empty grab you have time. With a full grab you have opportunity.

An easy rule to remember is "the rule of thumb." The thumb is the weak point of the hand. To escape almost any grab, simply **push, don't pull**, toward your opponent's wrist. This action will take their balance off guard if nothing else. If you find a greater resistance than you can conquer in this manner, think of your hand as a snake climbing and circling up a branch (your attacker's arm) and continuing on.

Additional Note: Leading is a common means by which you allow a grab with the intention of altering or controlling it, like letting the attacker grab you so you can throw him off balance.

Cross-handed Wrist Grab

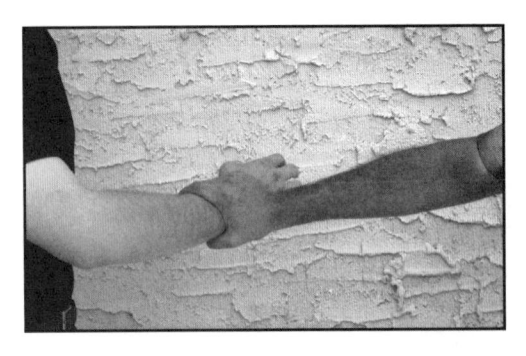

1. THE ATTACKER GRABS YOU WITH HIS CROSS HAND.

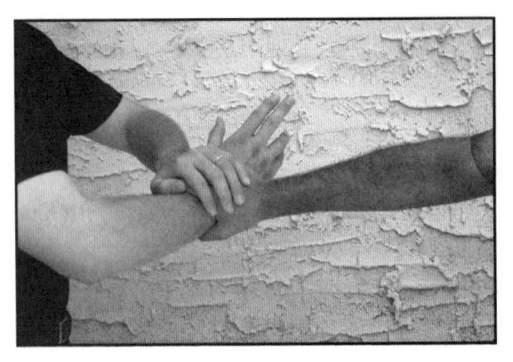

2. WITH YOUR FREE HAND, PRESS THE BASE OF YOUR PALM FIRMLY AGAINST YOUR ATTACKER'S FINGERTIPS.

LOCKS, GRAPPLING AND FREEING

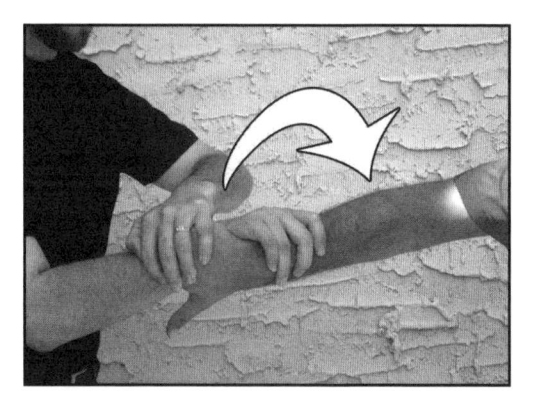

3. CURL YOUR MIRROR HAND FROM UNDERNEATH THE GRAB, TWISTING IT OVER THE SIDE OF THEIR WRIST.

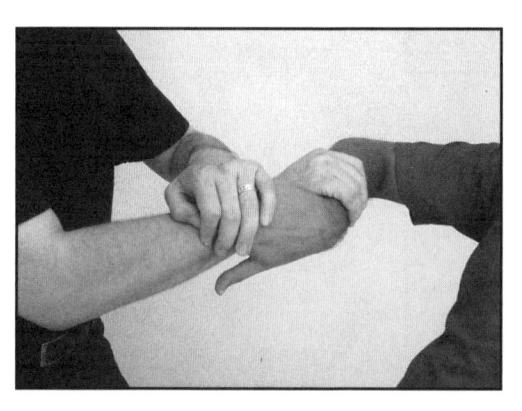

4. FORCE PRESSURE OVER THE SIDE OF THE WRIST UNTIL THE OPPONENT IS COMPLETELY UNDER CONTROL.

FULL BODY VIEW OF STEP 4

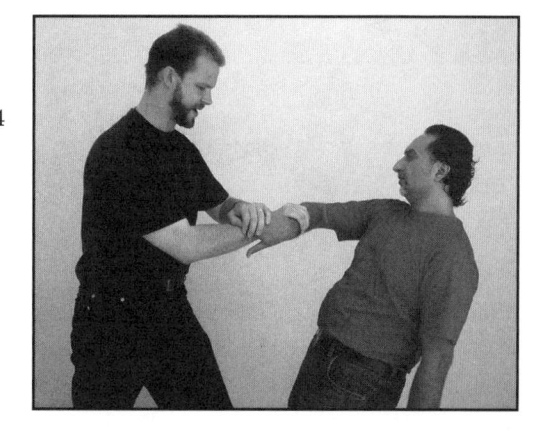

LOCKS, GRAPPLING AND FREEING

Mirror Handed Wrist Grab

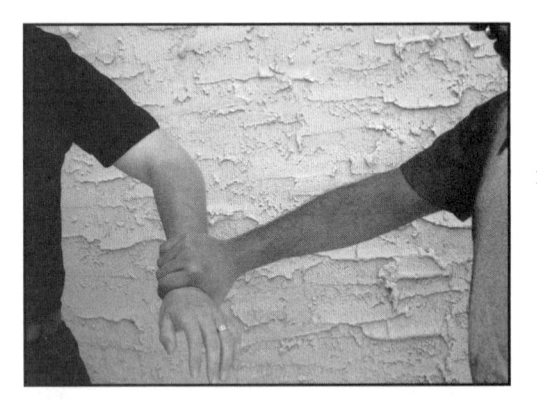

1. THE ATTACKER GRABS YOU WITH HIS MIRROR HAND.

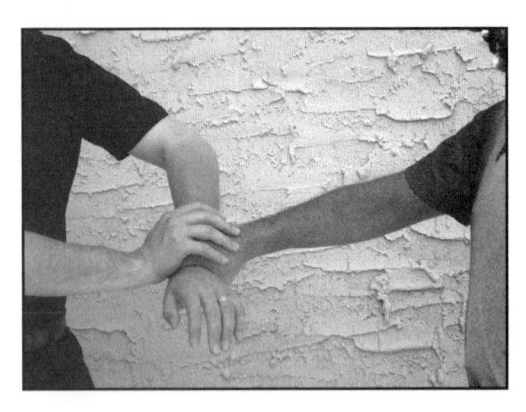

2. WITH YOUR FREE HAND, PRESS THE BASE OF YOUR PALM FIRMLY AGAINST YOUR ATTACKER'S FINGERTIPS.

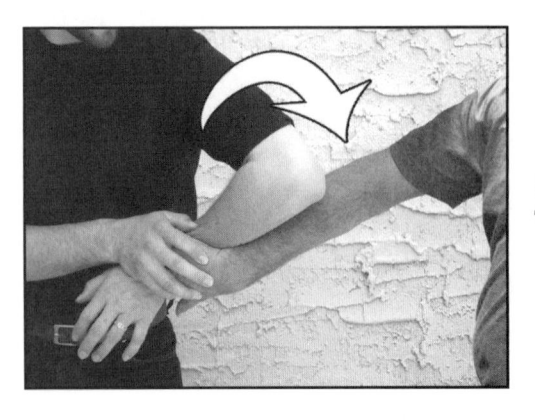

3. HOOK YOUR MIRROR ELBOW OVER THE SIDE OF THE ATTACKER'S WRIST.

LOCKS, GRAPPLING AND FREEING

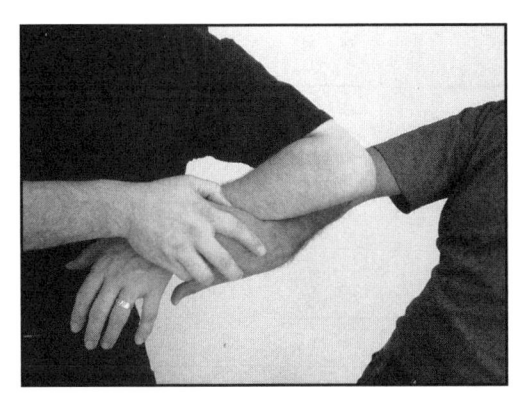

4. Force pressure over the side of wrist until the opponent is completely under control.

Full body view of Step 4

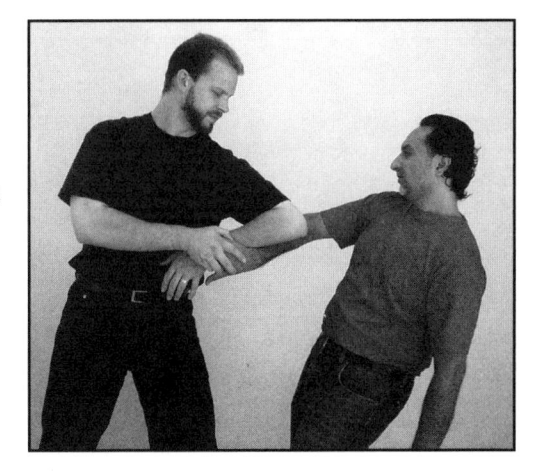

143

Quick Change Wrist Grab (High)

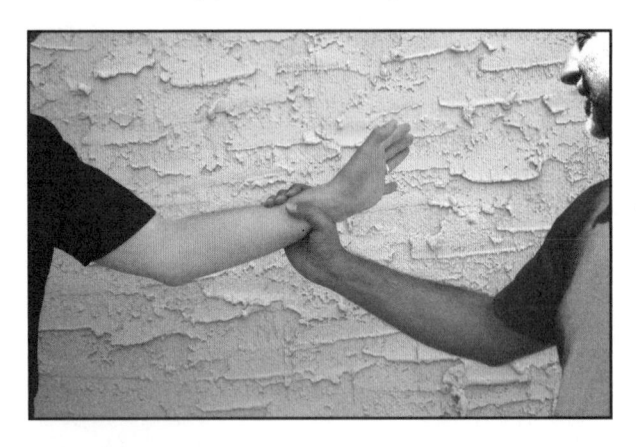

1. THE ATTACKER GRABS YOUR HAND AT THE WRIST FROM UNDERNEATH.

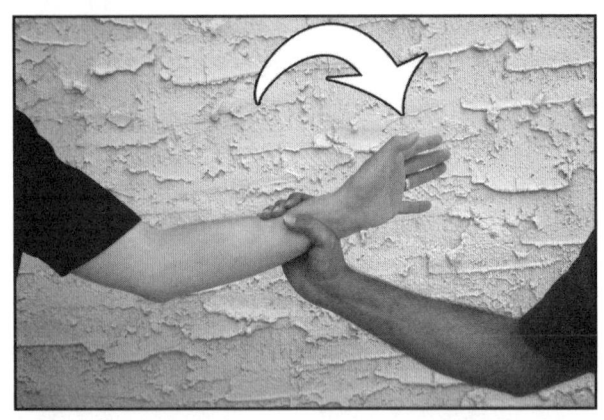

2. BEGIN POINTING YOUR FINGERS DOWN TOWARD THE WRIST OF THE ATTACKING HAND.

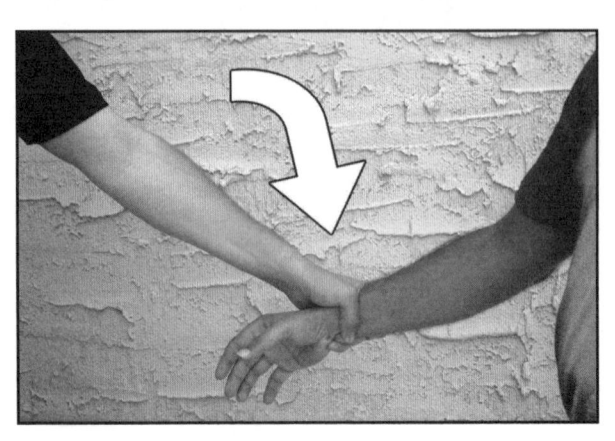

3. QUICKLY FORCE YOUR OWN GRAB OVER THE ATTACKER'S WRIST. DUE TO THE WEAKNESS OF THUMBS, YOUR ATTACKER WILL NOT BE ABLE TO MAINTAIN HIS HOLD.

LOCKS, GRAPPLING AND FREEING

Quick Change Wrist Grab (Low)

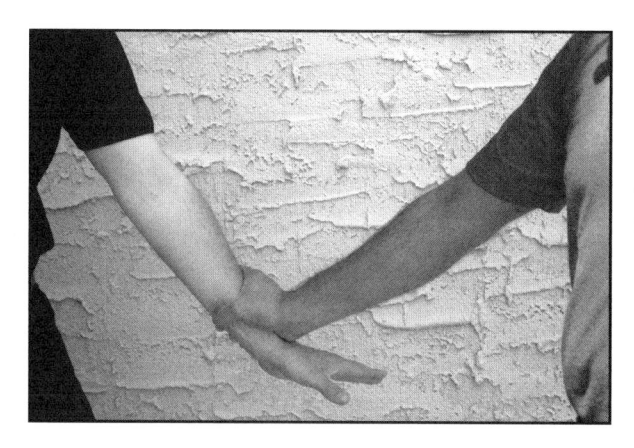

1. THE ATTACKER GRABS YOUR HAND AT THE WRIST FROM OVER THE TOP.

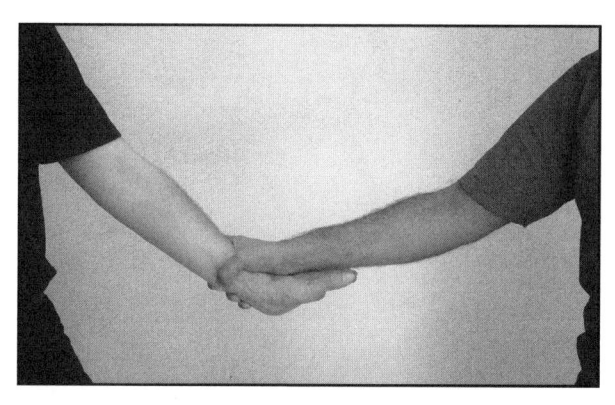

2. BEGIN POINTING YOUR FINGERS UP TOWARD THE WRIST OF THE ATTACKING HAND.

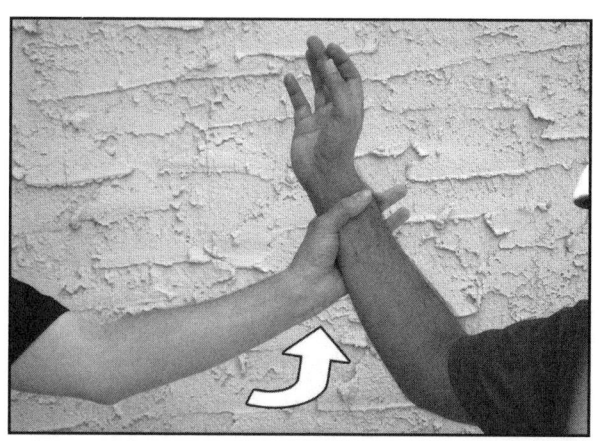

3. QUICKLY FORCE YOUR OWN GRAB UNDER THE ATTACKER'S WRIST. DUE TO THE WEAKNESS OF THUMBS, YOUR ATTACKER WILL NOT BE ABLE TO MAINTAIN THE HOLD.

STEPPING, TRAPPING AND FREEING

CHAPTER 7
STEPPING, TRAPPING and SWEEPS

One of the best pieces of advice that I have ever received came on my first night of bouncing. Having witnessed the tail-end of a fight including one of the more experienced members of the security team, I watched the offender being dragged away while one of the other bouncers held a metal pipe the offender had used in his attack. When I asked my colleague how he had left the fight unscathed, he stated that he had "Hit him with something even bigger." Seeing no weapon in sight, I asked his meaning. To answer this question, he told me to consider the largest object that I could hit someone with, such as a bat. After naming this, I was told to think of any one thing larger than that; perhaps a wooden door. He made me do this over and over again, making the objects larger each time until I came to the unavoidable solution, he had hit the attacker with the world itself. After this short explanation, I understood completely.

Gravity is the strongest force that any fighter can utilize. Any strike performed by a human being, no matter how strong they are, is grossly less than the simple force of gravity. Consider that your opponent weighs 180 lbs. If they fall, perhaps on their head, consider how that directly equates to 180 lbs of force, plus momentum, driving their fragile skull into the ground. A swift descent onto concrete is far less forgiving than the human fist. Most of the time, you will find that the majority of damage to your assailant will be incurred from the fall instead of the strike which caused it. With that in mind, we now analyze Stepping, Trapping, & Sweeps.

Stepping & Trapping

Stepping and trapping are achieved by denying movement to your opponent's legs and feet. Consider how simple a fight would be if your attacker lacked the ability to move from one specific place. However unrealistic an idea this might seem to be, with simple but specific foot placements we can "help" our attackers to achieve exactly that. By pinning our attackers to the ground, we can greatly limit their opportunities to deal us any harm.

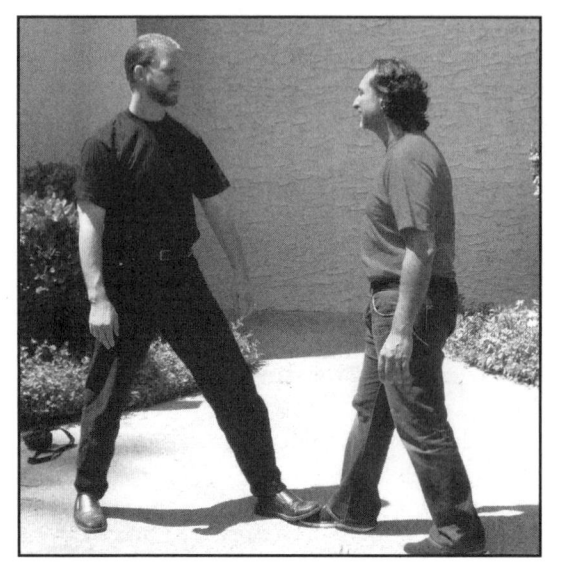

1. FIRMLY PRESS YOUR FOOT OVER YOUR OPPONENT'S TOES, PINNING THEM TO THE GROUND.

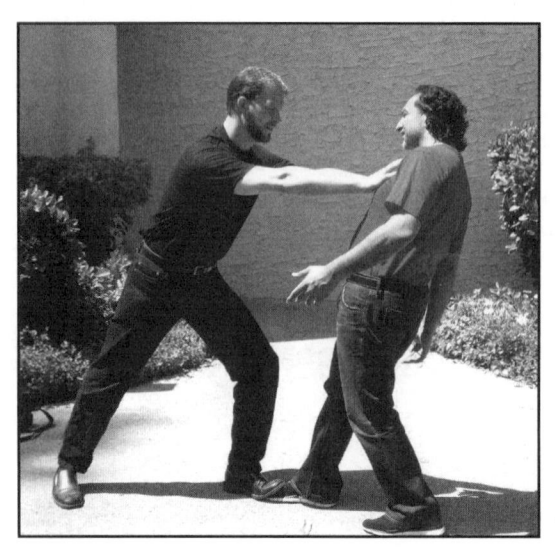

2. TRAP YOUR OPPONENT BY MAINTAINING THE FOOT PIN WHILE PUSHING YOUR OPPONENT BACKWARD.

Special note: Maintaining a foot trap after a push will tear the ligaments of the attacker's instep.

Sweeps

Sweeps are defined as any leg movement that upsets or alters your opponent's stability. Regardless of which is chosen, knocking your opponent off balance can be a very simple task if proper techniques are observed. First of all, you must consider your opponent's center of gravity. The entire weight of the human body is held up by two supporting limbs. Having said this, all one needs to do is remove the stability provided by one or both of the legs. The first manner in which to achieve this is to immobilize the support and move the body itself. The second is by removing the supporting limbs from beneath the body.

As stated previously in this chapter, gravity is the strongest force that any fighter can utilize. Any who believe differently should attempt to jump up and stay up without yielding to it's power. A quick and decisive victory can be gained by redirecting your energy or by simply using your opponent's own energy against him. Either will allow you to easily let them fall to this unforgiving natural force.

Cross Leg Sweep

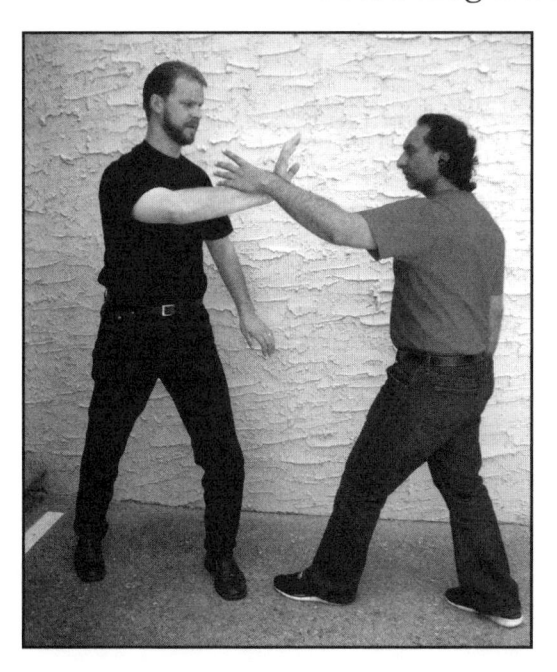

1. BLOCK THE OPPONENT'S ATTACK AT THE INNER WRIST WITH YOUR MIRROR HAND.

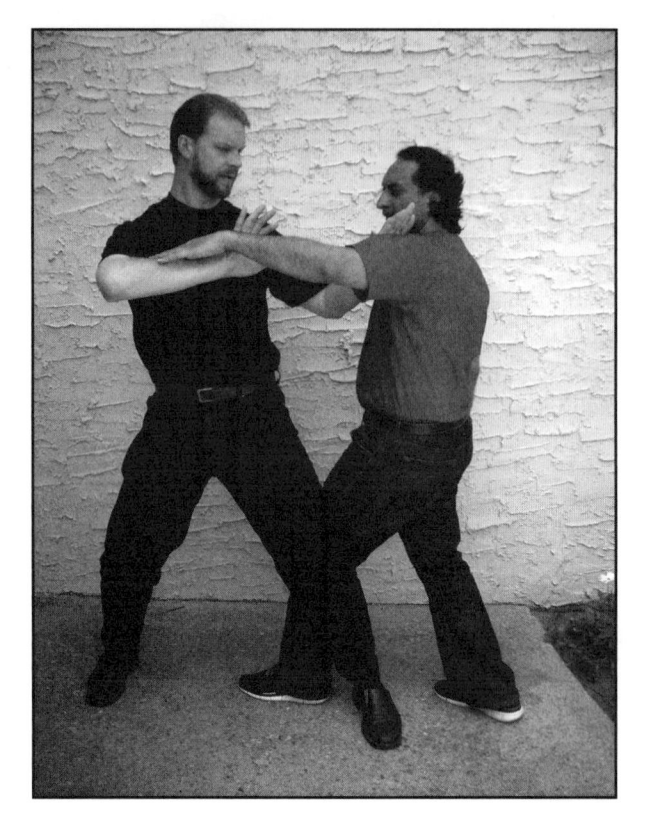

2. Step forward and behind his cross leg, while your cross hand presses the inside of the attacking shoulder.

STEPPING, TRAPPING AND FREEING

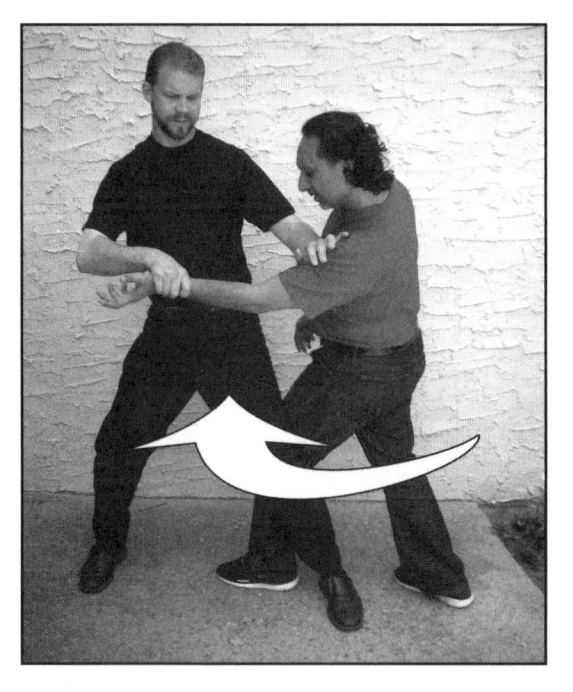

3A. TWIST YOUR HIPS TO THROW ATTACKER TO THE GROUND.

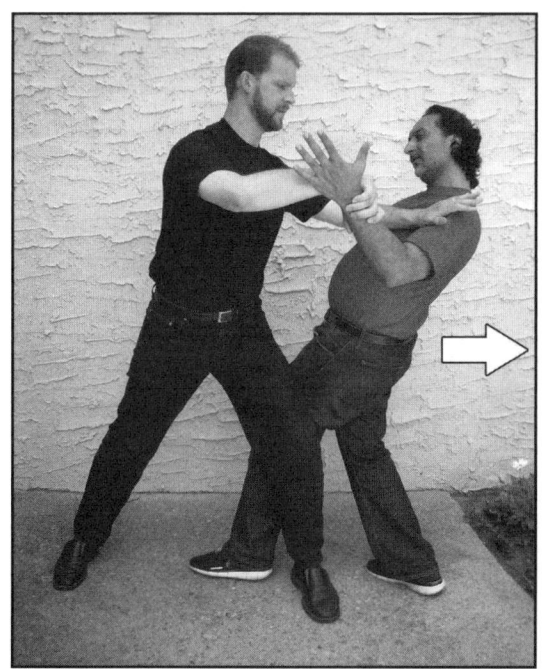

OR

3B. PRESS BACKWARD TO THROW ATTACKER TO THE GROUND.

Mirror Leg Sweep

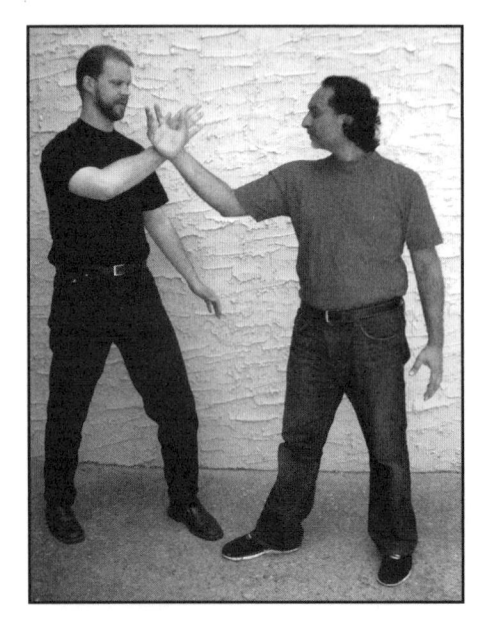

1. Block the cross handed attack at the wrist.

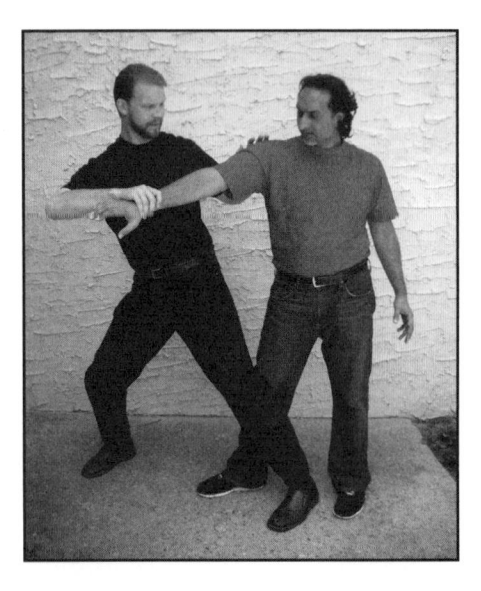

2. Stepping in front of the attacker with your mirror foot, placing your mirror hand on the outside of the attacking shoulder.

STEPPING, TRAPPING AND FREEING

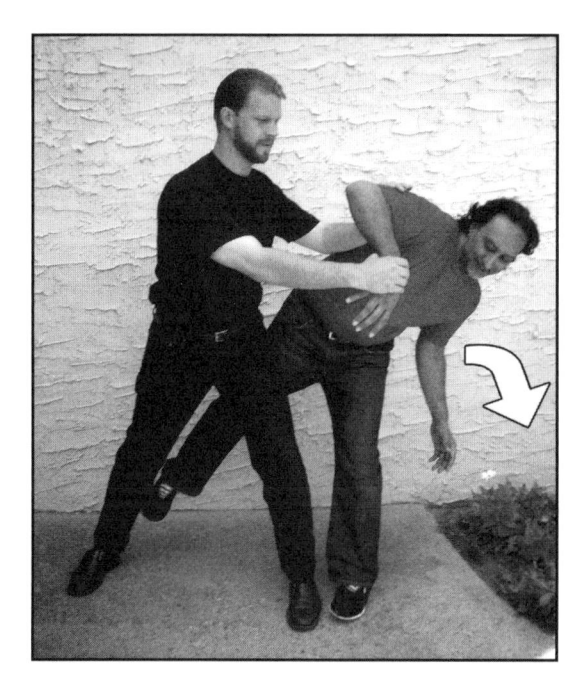

3A. Twist your hips to throw the attacker to the ground.

OR

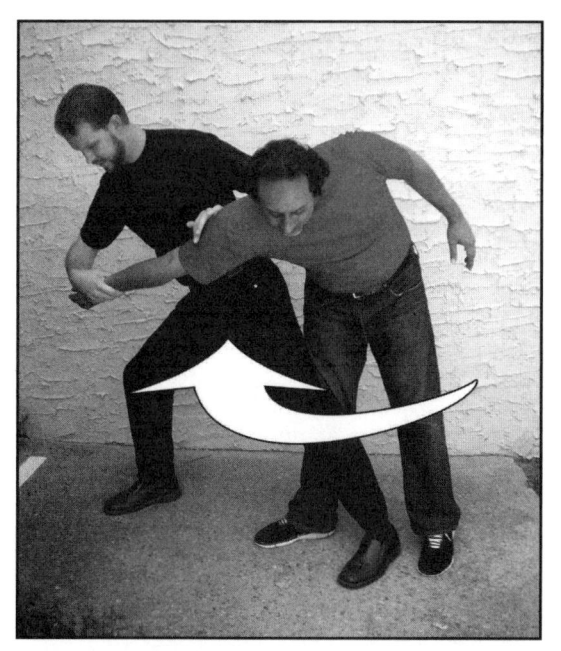

3B. Press forward to throw the attacker to the ground.

READING YOUR OPPONENT

CHAPTER 8
READING YOUR OPPONENT

Most martial arts techniques are simple, it's just that the average person would never think of them. That is not to say that mastery is easy, but rather that aptitude is attainable to any who seek it. Considering a few characteristics of your opponent can read volumes into them. Observe their movement or lack thereof. Recognize favoring or leaning. Once in battle, determine if they are they an "in" or "out" fighter. Identify if they offer a recurrence of the same attack. These are only a few of the insights you will gain from this section.

The purpose of this final chapter is to show you exactly how to spot your attacker's openings and weaknesses. After reading, you will be armed with the knowledge of how to render any attack useless before it has even been attempted.

Unfortunately, there are two things that no teacher can grant to a student, experience and confidence. Those each fighter must gain on his/her own. Remember that training is essential to competence with any system. Practice randomly. You need not be in battle with someone to take the opportunity to read them. With every customer, man or woman, that walked into the club, I monitored each person's movement, checking to see if I could find a tell of aggression or anger. Most experienced bouncers are never surprised by the persons in the club who start the fights. If fact, the reason for our own very successful team was that we all informed each other of potential aggressors, keeping a close eye on them throughout the night. By the time anyone started a skirmish, almost every bouncer in the club knew of their location, how much they had to drink, their companions, and any other physical determinations that presented themselves. These preparations will become second nature to you and the more you practice, the greater your ability will be. When considering preemptive movement, think of the old adage, "It takes a second to learn, A lifetime to master."

Preemptive Movement

Situations arise where you know that you are in danger. A drunkard ranting loudly at you while holding a broken beer bottle in his hand is an absolute, but it is unfortunately not always this obvious. Most times your opponent will try to hide their intentions from you, assuming the element of surprise will win them the fight. Such was the case of one patron I remember who pretended to ignore my presence while cupping a hidden knife in his hand. Had it not been for my training in Diamond Point Fighting (see Chapter 1) and a brief glimmer of light that bounced off of the blade from one of the dance floor lights, that situation might have ended quite differently. However, having seen the glint reflect off of his weapon and knowing the threat was absolute, I prepared myself.

Once you feel certain that your situation is nothing less than dangerous to your physical wellbeing, such as when verbal or physical threats have been made, you should prepare. Consider though, preemptive movement does not limit itself to being performed solely at the onset of an altercation, but rather it can be use at any point during a fight. For example, if you are attacked from behind, free yourself, create a distance, and then perform the techniques of preemptive movement to secure your safety.

Once again I must reiterate, these sequences and techniques are ONLY to be used when you know that grave physical harm is certain and imminent. Use the techniques wrongfully and you may find yourself behind bars for an unprovoked assault. Remember that there is a great difference between persons who are willing assailants and those whom we are simply wary of.

If you do, however, find yourself with knowledge of an oncoming attack, consider the game of chess. Defeating your assailant can happen several steps before an attack is even made. Reading your opponent and analyzing their stance, movement, posture, etc., can grant you the knowledge of how to conquer them before they come within several feet of you.

Observe the distance your opponent is from you. Knowing that every pace covers about 2 1/2 feet, gauge how many steps it will take for them to reach you. Your goal is to measure how many paces they must take before they are upon you and be ready to jump in before their last step. If your opponent is 3 paces away, be ready to move in over the landing of their second step.

READING YOUR OPPONENT

Preemptive Movement Reading

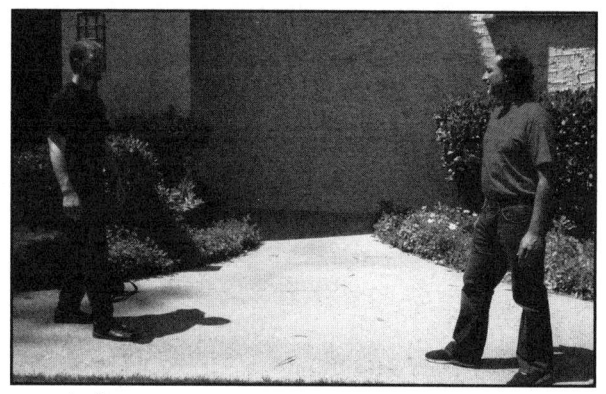

1. Opponent stands ready 3 paces from you.

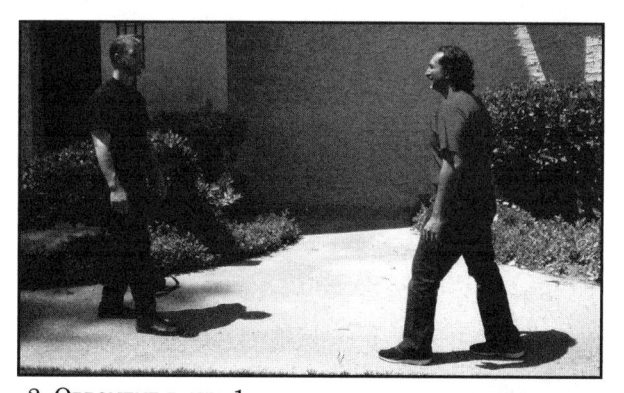

2. Opponent takes 1st step toward you agressively.

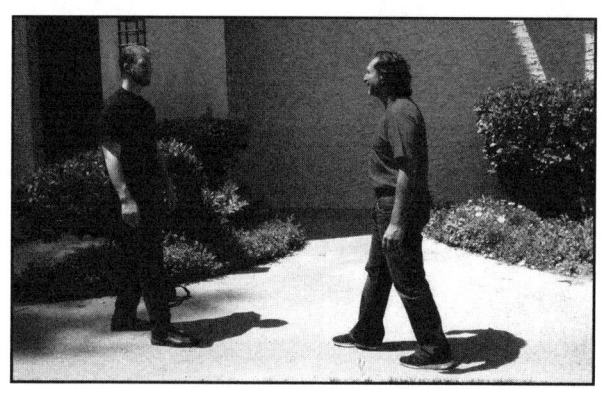

3. Opponent takes 2nd step.

READING YOUR OPPONENT

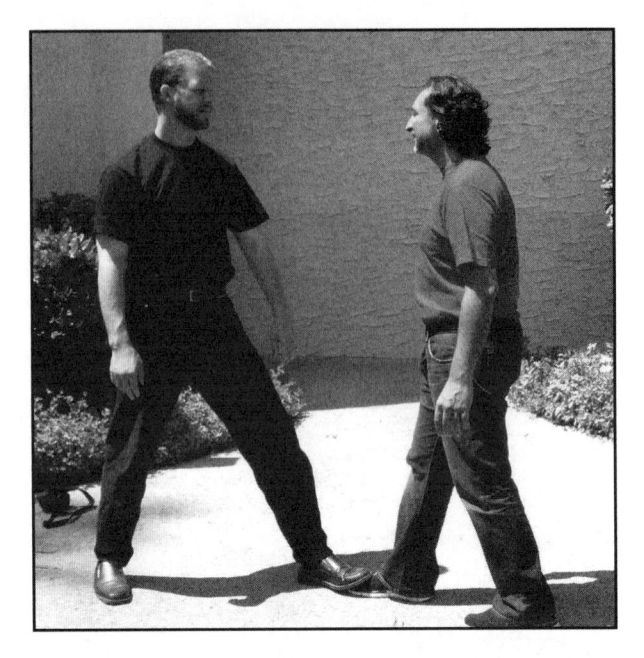

4. Before the opponent can take a 3rd step, move forward, stepping atop the foot which just landed. It is very important to attack the non-stepping foot.

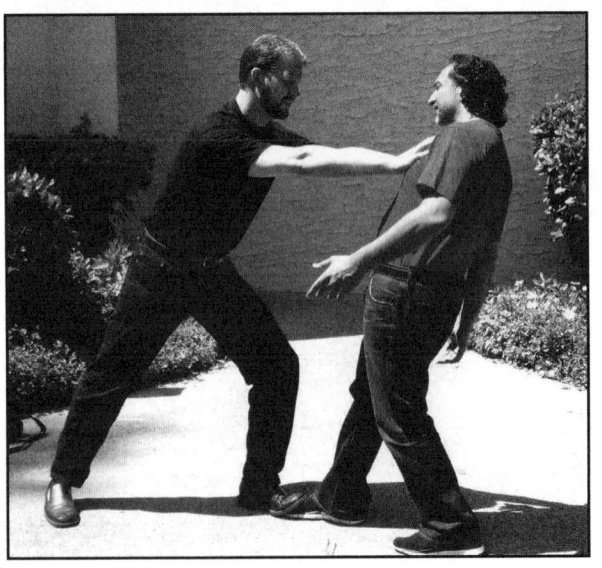

5. Maintaining pressure over foot, press against attacker, forcing him to the ground.

Stances

Recognize the system of fighting your attacker plans to utilize and you will have a functioning knowledge of the skills they will use. Below are a few of the more broad stance representations. Considering the techniques of each and how a fighter would use them will grant you a look into the weaknesses and strengths for each. By recognizing your opponent's stance, certain hypotheses can be achieved (as listed below).

Martial Arts Stance

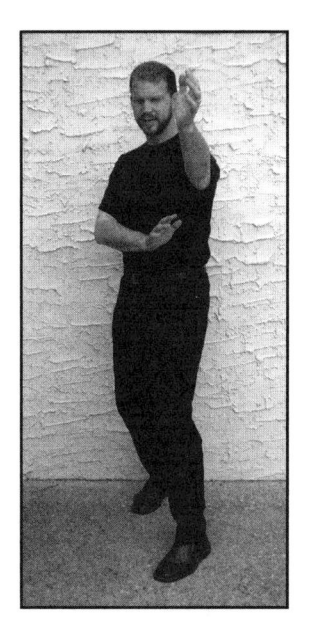

1. The fighter is certainly prepared to use kicks as well as punches.

2. The "center-line," (Throat, Heart, Groin) is turned to the side, leaving the back, (Spine, Lungs, Kidneys) as viable options.

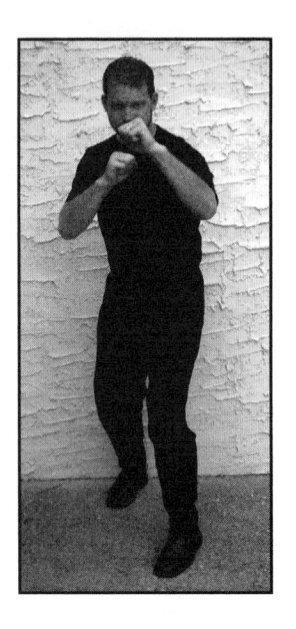

Boxing Stance

1. The fighter will probably rely on upper body attacks.

2. The fighter is almost certainly used to taking strikes to the head and torso, but not to the lower body.

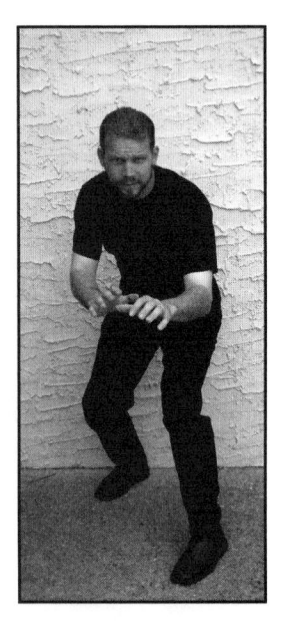

Grappling Stance

1. The fighter will almost certainly not limit their attack to punches and kicks.

2. The fighter will readily take the fight to the ground and may not be comfortable with standing to fight.

Guarding Postures

Reading your opponent is not only limited to recognizing their preference, but also their well-being. Spotting an injury or weakness can be as easy as viewing the level and position of your attacker's blocking. Below are listed a few common ailments.

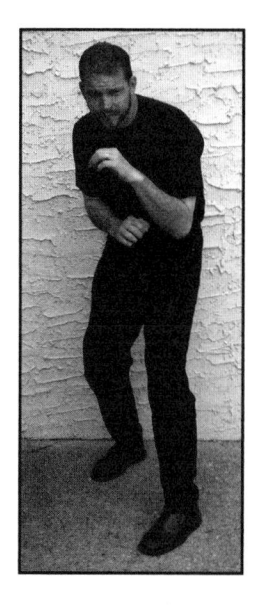

STOMACH GUARDING POSTURE

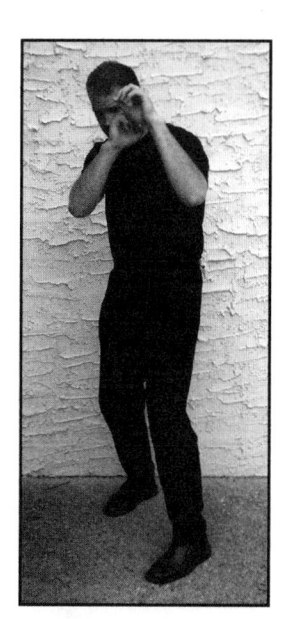

FACE GUARDING POSTURE

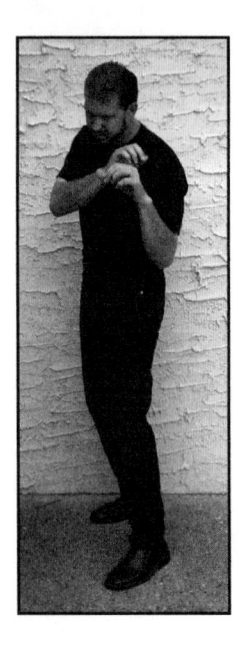

RIBCAGE GUARDING POSTURE

Summary

Defending oneself is not a difficult thing. Remember that your own personal safety, and not bravado, comes first. Be wise, calm, and patient. Follow the simple rules outlined in this guide, practice them, and you will have gained knowledge that will protect you in any situation.

About the Author

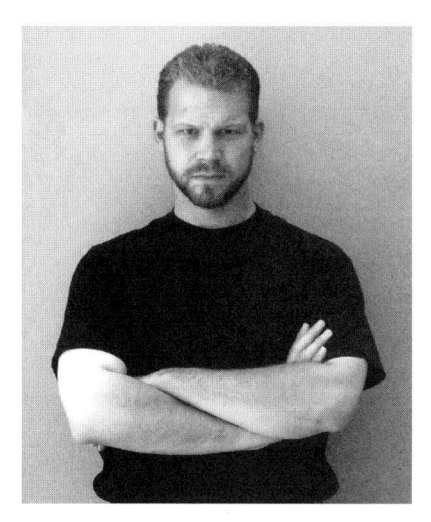

Sifu Noah Knapp has over 24 years experience in the martial arts. He has a 3rd degree black sash in Northern Drunken Style Kung Fu as well as training in Kenpo, Karate, Aikido, Kali, Silat & Tai Chi. He is a 2nd generation instructor at his family's kung fu school as well as an instructor for the STAR martial arts program. He has had the opportunity to advance his knowledge in real-life situations, serving as head of security and/or bouncer at many Los Angeles nightclubs including: The Playroom, A.D., The Gate, The Lounge and Balboa. You can contact him at sifunoah@yahoo.com.

Index

#

3 point destruction rolling fists 69
3 point downward rolling fists 67–68
3 point Inside rolling fists 63–64
3 point outside rolling fists 61–62
3 point rolling fists 60–69
3 point upward rolling fists 65–66
4 point bridge rolling fists 74–75
4 point destruction rolling fists 78–79
4 point downward rolling fists 76–77
4 point inside rolling fists 72–73
4 point outside rolling fists 70–71
4 point rolling fists 70–79

A

acute elbow strike 54–55
arm attacks 48–51
arm bar 136–139

B

backfist 28–29
backward facing headlock 127–129
back kick 102–103
ball of foot attack 97
bear hug 134–135
bent joint 13
block 60, 113
boxing stance 160
brush-by attack 52
bump separation 93

C

center-line 159
check kick 121
chop 44, 46–47
claw strike 40–41
closed hand attacks 22
close combat 48, 95, 123
cross-handed wrist grab 140

cross hand 59

D

defense 60
destruction 54
diamond points 14–19
double handed choke 132–133
double handed push 88–89
double hand tunneling 81–83

E

eagle's beak 32–33
elbow strikes 52–56
empty grab 140
energy 57, 60, 149

F

finger gouge 34–35
finishing strikes 60
fist 23, 24
flying kick 112
forearm strike 50–51
forward facing headlock 124–126
forward pullback 86–87
front kick 99–100
full grab 140
full nelson 130–131

G

grabbing 113
grappling 123
grappling stance 160
gravity 147, 149
Guarding posture 161–162

H

half fist 26–27
hand attacks 21, 24–47
headlocks 124–133

heart strike 38
heel Attack 96
high-level kick 111–112
high-level knee attack 106
high kicks 95, 111

I

instep attack 97

J

jump kick 112

K

kicks 95–96, 99–105
kick separation 91
knee attacks 106–108, 118–120
knife hand 44–45
knuckle fist 30–31
knuckle rake 30

L

locked joint 13
low-level knee attack 108
low kicks 121
low level leg attacks 121

M

manipulation 90
martial arts stance 159
mastery 155
mid-level leg attack 113–120
midsection 26
mirror hand 58
mirror handed wrist grab 142–143
mirror leg sweep 152–153

O

obtuse elbow strike 52–53
offense 60
openings 155

P

palm strike 38–39
poke 34

posture 12
preemptive movement 155–158
pressure point 32, 36
pulling 113
punch 22, 24–25, 60
push position 80
push separation 92

Q

quick change wrist grab 144–145

R

reading your opponent 155
ready stance 12–13
rolling fists 57, 69–79

S

scanning 16
separations 91–93
side kick 104–105
single hand entry 84–85
slap 42
soft strike 23, 40
spreading waves 88–89
stability 149
stances 159–160
star fist 32–33
stepping and trapping 148
sweeps 149–153

T

thumb spike 36–37
touch sensitivity 80
training 155
tunneling 80–90

U

upper body attacks 22

W

ward off position 12–13, 113
whip hand 42–43
wrist grab 140–145
wrist strike 48–49

Also Available from Turtle Press:

Boxing: Advanced Tactics and Strategies
Vital Leglocks
Grappler's Guide to Strangles and Chokes
Fighter's Fact Book 2
The Armlock Encyclopedia
Championship Sambo
Complete Taekwondo Poomse
Martial Arts Injury Care and Prevention
Timing for Martial Arts
Strength and Power Training
Complete Kickboxing
Ultimate Flexibility
Boxing: A 12 Week Course
The Fighter's Body: An Owner's Manual
The Science of Takedowns, Throws and Grappling for Self-defense
Fighting Science
Martial Arts Instructor's Desk Reference
Solo Training
Solo Training 2
Fighter's Fact Book
Conceptual Self-defense
Martial Arts After 40
Warrior Speed
The Martial Arts Training Diary for Kids
Teaching Martial Arts
Combat Strategy
The Art of Harmony
Total MindBody Training
1,001 Ways to Motivate Yourself and Others
Ultimate Fitness through Martial Arts
Taekwondo Kyorugi: Olympic Style Sparring

For more information:
Turtle Press
1-800-77-TURTL
e-mail: orders@turtlepress.com

http://www.turtlepress.com